The Foundation Programme for Doctors

The Foundation Programme for Doctors

Getting in, getting on and getting out

Ferras Alwan
Undertaking an intercalated BSc between fourth and final years of medicine at Barts and the London, Queen Mary's School of Medicine and Dentistry, London

Rohin Francis MBBS, BSc (Hons)
FY1 doctor, St Peter's Hospital, Chertsey, Surrey
Graduated June 2006 from St George's Hospital Medical School, London

and

Emma-Jane Smith BSc (Hons)
Penultimate-year medical student at Royal Free and University College Medical School, University College London, London

Foreword by

Jane Dacre
Academic Vice President, Royal College of Physicians of London
Vice Dean and Professor of Medical Education, Royal Free & University College Medical School, University College London
Consultant Physician and Rheumatologist

Radcliffe Publishing
Oxford • Seattle

Radcliffe Publishing Ltd
18 Marcham Road
Abingdon
Oxon OX14 1AA
United Kingdom

www.radcliffe-oxford.com
Electronic catalogue and worldwide online ordering facility.

_____

Reprinted 2007

British Library Cataloguing in Publication Data

A catalogue record for this book is available from the British Library.

ISBN-10: 1 84619 116 5
ISBN-13: 978 1 84619 116 9

Typeset by Aarontype Ltd, Easton, Bristol
Printed and bound by TJI Digital, Padstow, Cornwall

Contents

About the authors

Ferras, Rohin and Emma-Jane have been the editors of *Medical Student Newspaper* (www.medical-student.co.uk) since its first full year of publication. Their commitment won the paper the title of 'Best Small Budget Publication' at the 2005 National Union of Students/*Daily Mirror* National Student Journalism Awards, and each of them holds a University of London Laurel Award for their work.

Ferras Alwan is currently undertaking an intercalated degree in community health sciences at Barts and the London, Queen Mary's School of Medicine and Dentistry, before entering his final year in 2007. He was nominated for Student Campaigner of the Year at the University of London Student Action Awards 2006 for his work on the Multi-Deanery Application Process (MDAP) as Deputy Chair of the University of London Union MedGroup.

Rohin Francis graduated from St George's Hospital Medical School in June 2006. He also holds an intercalated BSc in basic medical sciences. Rohin scored 42/48 on his MDAP form, making him one of the top scorers in the UK and securing him his first-choice Foundation year 1 post at St Peter's Hospital, Chertsey.

Emma-Jane Smith is in her penultimate year at the Royal Free and University College Medical School, University College London (UCL). She holds an intercalated BSc in physiology and a Merit in medical sciences. In 2006 she was awarded UCL Union Centenary Colours for her dedication to *Medical Student Newspaper* and the student community of UCL.

Foreword

The implementation of Modernising Medical Careers will be recognised as a very good thing in retrospect. At the time of writing, it is still a source of great anxiety to the doctors responsible for its delivery, and to those who will be going through it. This book will help to allay that anxiety by explaining the Foundation Years, and the rationale behind the change.

This book will be an invaluable resource for our new generation of doctors. It takes readers through the process from application, to F2 and beyond. It offers useful advice in a useable and readable format. It is written by a group of current and past medical students who have lived through, and continue to live through, the insecurities of the changing medical career structures. Its style is informal, engaging and easy to absorb, so it should be a good distraction for those currently in the run-up to their finals exams. Good luck to all of you, and don't forget, Medicine is a wonderful career.

Jane Dacre
Academic Vice President, Royal College of Physicians of London
Vice Dean and Professor of Medical Education,
Royal Free & University College Medical School,
University College London
Consultant Physician and Rheumatologist
January 2007

For my mum and dad.
FA

For Mum, Neil and June.
RF

For Ginnie and Charlie, to whom I owe all my successes.
EJS

We are sincerely grateful to the whole team at Radcliffe Publishing for their advice and support in producing this book but would like to specifically thank Suse Rabson, who was instrumental in helping us create it and without whom it never would have been written. Thanks Suse!

Chapter 1

Overview of Modernising Medical Careers and the Foundation Programme

Introduction

Once upon a time, there was a girl called Hannah. Now Hannah was a bright girl and liked helping people, so she decided that she wanted to be a doctor. She went to medical school, worked very hard for five years and at the end became Dr Hannah. Dr Hannah liked medical school a lot, especially all the blood and gore, so she decided she wanted to be a trauma surgeon. She completed her pre-registration house officer (PRHO) year, worked as a senior house officer (SHO) for three years and as a registrar for four years, then got a job as a consultant in a prestigious London teaching hospital, married a semi-literate footballer and lived happily ever after.

Although people have always perceived this to be the way progression in medical careers happens, it is in fact a myth. Climbing the job ladder in medicine has always been a messy affair, and certainly not something for the faint-hearted. For one thing, it never happened as easily as in Hannah's case. In theory you only worked as an SHO for three or four years, but the reality was that this was the minimum. You applied for jobs that often had 1,000 other candidates going for them, so you can imagine jobs didn't often go to the plucky young SHO applying for the first time. As a result, it is not uncommon to hear stories of people who have done five, six or even seven years as an SHO. And if you think you're sorted once you become a registrar and have picked up your National Training Number then think again, because the whole scenario repeats itself – complete your training and then apply for jobs over and over and over again until you finally get lucky.

All in all, it was a long, hard graft, and so it was decided that postgraduate training needed to change. And what a change it was! Modernising Medical Careers, commonly abbreviated to MMC, is probably the biggest change in medicine since the NHS started. It is big, and when we say big, we mean BIG. We're talking *New Coke* replacing Classic Coca-Cola big; we're talking Peter Crouch standing on Jan Koller's shoulders big; we're talking double-quarter-pounder with cheese, mayo, salad, bacon, fried egg and a hash brown all in a sesame bun, with a side order of large fries, onion rings, a double deluxe coke and an apple pie to finish. That's how big it is. Remember when *The Fresh Prince of Bel-Air* replaced the actress who played Vivian? It's even bigger than that. This is a fundamental change to how everything is done in medicine, and it's going to affect everyone currently in medical school.

Modernising Medical Careers

MMC came about as a result of a 2002 consultation paper called *Unfinished Business*, written by the Chief Medical Officer, Sir Liam Donaldson. Now

Sir Liam wasn't too happy with the way postgraduate medical training in the UK was working. In particular, he was worried about senior house officers. SHOs make up half of all training doctors in the UK, but have long had to make do with the short end of the stick. To begin with, even the statement 'SHOs are half of all training doctors' is in fact a misnomer, because almost half of these posts were dead-end jobs/short-term appointments that were not part of any training programme. And across the whole board, there was a lack of careers advice to make sure you were on the right track to do what you wanted to do. The problems with the SHO grade didn't end there. A big issue was that the quality of the jobs varied wildly. Some firms could be amazing, teaching you everything you needed to know to be the world's best SHO. Others weren't so good and you could find yourself having to make do with little or no teaching in subjects that were of no use to you, and with no methods of assessing whether or not you knew all that you should. There was very little option for flexibility in your training and, as we've already mentioned, there was no guarantee how many years you'd have to work before you were accepted into specialist training.

So Sir Liam proposed some changes to the grade. First of all, he wanted to get rid of the issue of different programmes being of different quality, so he suggested that rules be set on how training would be delivered. This would accompany a programme curriculum that would set out what an SHO needed to know. All of this would culminate in what had previously been a novel concept – quality assurance of training. Doctors would be tested on this knowledge by assessments that were consistent wherever you worked and whatever specialty you were working in. The training would be broadly based, so no matter what SHO job you did, it would equip you with the skills necessary to move into your desired specialty. There would be a time-cap to it all, so no more waiting around for seven years before you progressed to specialist training. (The latter point sounds great, but it goes hand in hand with another principle of reform that what the NHS needs in terms of specialists, and what doctors want to be, are not necessarily the same thing, but more on this later.) Finally, the changing demographics of medicine were taken into consideration, and with the majority of medical students carrying two copies of the X chromosome, *Unfinished Business* proposed that there should be more opportunities for flexible training to ensure that things like wanting a family wouldn't disadvantage trainees.

So, armed with all of these recommendations made by the Nation's Doctor™, the powers that be got together and designed MMC. Now if you've been following so far, you'll probably agree that the basic premise of MMC sounds reasonable enough – postgraduate training is a long, hard slog, demoralising to those in it and not producing enough doctors in the right specialties for the public. The solution to this? A complete overhaul of postgraduate medical training.

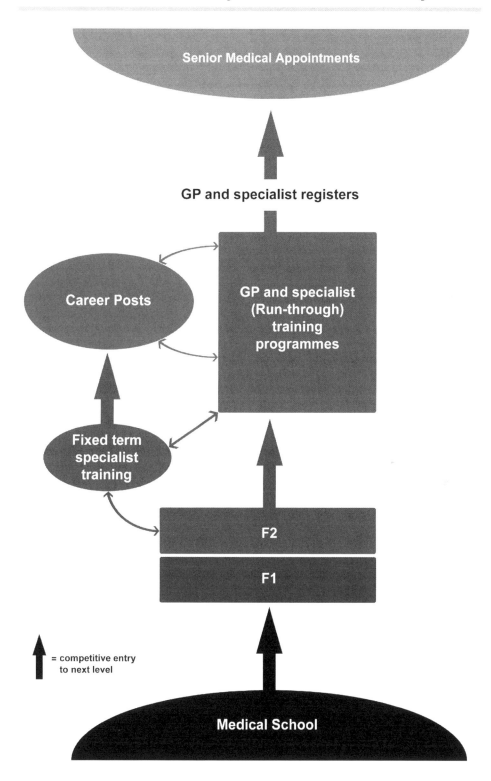

Figure 1.1.

The new structure to postgraduate training

As mentioned earlier, the lack of a clear pathway of progression was one of the main problems with the old training grade. The answer to this problem was to devise a streamlined scheme whereby doctors move from one stage to the next in a continuous flow without hanging about. A medical career will now start with a two-year Foundation Programme. This is subdivided into foundation year 1 (FY1) and foundation year 2 (FY2), and both will last for precisely one year – no more, no less. FY1 will still be a pre-registration year, and successful completion of it will be needed before the General Medical Council (GMC) add you to their list of registered medical practitioners. FY1 posts are only open to those who have not previously worked as a doctor anywhere in the world, but FY2 posts are open to all. On completion of FY2, doctors will immediately move into specialist training. This is one of the big changes – it's no longer a case of 'you're now eligible, so start applying for posts', as was the case with the old SHO grade. It's now 'you've finished your foundation training, so bugger off!' You will have to move into specialist training, and although in theory this sounds like a good idea, it also causes one of the biggest problems of MMC. You see, in the old system, a lot of the waiting was self-inflicted – doctors waited around for years because they were hoping to be a plastic surgeon and there were only a few training jobs out there in that field. That's undoubtedly a pain, but at least you got to do the job that really interested you once you finally entered specialist training. No such luck in the MMC world. Once you finish your specialist training you will be faced with two options.

1 Apply for specialist training posts, and if you don't get the one of your choice make do with whatever specialties are left at the end of it all.
2 Decide that you only want to work in one field and if you don't get a place on a training scheme, follow that specialty in a non-training grade, the so-called 'career grades'.

A word about career grades. This new and enticing moniker should be approached with caution. Non-training grades were formerly known as career-grade doctors or trust doctors, and these posts were regarded as career suicide. Once you took such a post, you could kiss your hopes of ever becoming a consultant or principal GP goodbye, because you'd be stuck there for the rest of your working life. They are posts created by trusts to fill specific shortages in their departments, and are not approved by postgraduate training deaneries, which means that you will never acquire the skills you need to move up the ladder. Even though MMC does say there will be a route of escape for those in career grades, it's still best to avoid these positions at all costs. That means you're best sticking to the specialist training path and taking whatever it throws at you, even if it's not exactly what you want. While one of the biggest attractions of a medical career has always been the diverse choice of jobs and the ability to specialise in the one that really grabs you, the thinking behind this change is logical enough. Specialties such as microbiology, psychiatry, histo-pathology and public health medicine are obviously crucial to the health service, but are not attracting enough applicants to their training schemes. Rather than providing the opportunity for everyone to train in the field of their choice and the UK ending up with thousands of plastic surgeons (and a much prettier population as a result, so it's not all bad!), the specialties available in specialist training will mirror the requirements of the population, so if there's an acute shortage of radiologists, the scheme will aim to churn out more of them.

There's another problem here, too. You're deciding your future career path after only two years in medicine, or more accurately a year and a half, because you'll be applying for specialist training posts halfway through FY2. This requires extreme focus on the part of the medical student/junior doctor. Next time you're on the ward, ask one of the registrars or consultants when they decided on their chosen specialty. The chances are they'll tell you that it was deep into their SHO training, probably after dabbling with two, three or maybe even four other career paths beforehand. Ask them whether they had any idea what they'd do when they were in medical school, or if they thought they'd be doing this back then. They will laugh at you. The reality is, in the post-MMC world, you're going to have to start thinking seriously about careers that interest you while you're still in medical school. Whether this is a good thing or a bad thing remains to be seen.

The make-up of the foundation years

The key word here is 'generic'. Whatever job you do, in whatever specialties, in whatever hospital in the UK, the theory is that you'll be learning the same things, as guided by the curriculum (more on this in Chapter 4). In each foundation year you'll do a mix of specialties in posts which can be 3, 4 or 6 months in length (but always a cumulative total of 12 months, so you could do three 4-month jobs, or two 6-month jobs, for example), and soon 90% of all Foundation Programmes will include general practice as one of the rotations. This is in line with the govern-ment's wishes for more doctors to become general practitioners because they see them as gatekeepers to the NHS, who can treat patients before their illness becomes serious and not refer them to expensive hospital beds.

In addition to this likely GP rotation, each programme will have a good mix of specialties, including at least one surgical post and as much expo-sure to emergency medicine as possible. The issue of specialties suffering from a shortage of doctors is addressed here, too. The aim is that as few

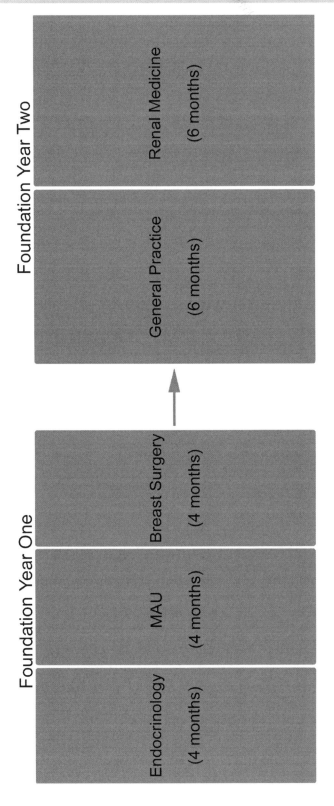

Figure 1.2.

people are forced to move into specialties that they don't like as possible, and rather that they will consider jobs that previously hadn't crossed their minds. This will be achieved by including the specialties that are perceived as 'less desirable' as part of many of the Foundation Programmes, and it looks as if it'll be a good idea. Certainly this was the case when the pilot programmes experimented with including a general practice rotation. A number of the trainees had no interest in it before they started the rotation, but changed their minds after they had tried it. Even those who had their minds set on other careers still said that they gained a lot from the experience and didn't regret it in the least. The theory is that this will work for other specialties, too. For example, many people are put off genito-urinary medicine by inaccurate preconceptions, but those who have worked in it find it a pretty satisfying career. Even if it doesn't catch your interest, it provides a good foundation of knowledge that is useful in other fields such as gynaecology and rheumatology. The posts that you do in the foundation years will have no impact whatsoever on the careers that you can apply to in specialist training, so it's to your advantage to experiment here and try specialties you'd not previously considered or that you know little about. Equally, the hospitals that you work in won't matter, so all those myths about how good it looks on your CV if you do your first job in a busy teaching hospital go straight out of the window. You might have your heart set on being a paediatric surgeon, but you never know – those three months in a district general hospital doing chemical pathology may come in very useful in the future!

Students will either apply to a full two-year Foundation Programme and so will know the make-up of both years in advance, or will initially apply only for FY1, and halfway through that will apply for FY2.

Specialist training

Once you've done your two foundation years, you move on to specialist training or 'run-through training' as it's now called. As with the foundation years, this will be for a fixed term, the length differing for each specialty. Each field of medicine will adhere to its own set curriculum to make sure that you learn everything you're meant to know. On completion you'll be awarded a CCT – a Certificate of Completion of Training. Get this baby and you'll be free to apply for consultant and principal GP jobs to your heart's content, right? Wrong again. Yes, you'll be applying for specialist posts, but they'll be under the banner of 'senior medical appointments', and to quote the MMC Career Framework directly, these can include 'GP principals, other employed GPs, consultants or *other specialist roles*. These roles will be determined by the service.' The worry here is that we'll end up with some kind of sub-consultant grade – doctors who have completed their specialist training but who can only work in specific areas, without the pay and privileges that are given to a 'full' consultant. With specialist training not due to even begin until August 2007, it will be a good few years before we find out more as to how true this will be.

Run-through training will be available in all specialties, but not every specialty will be available in every part of the UK. Obviously, the major specialties like orthopaedics and paediatrics will have programmes all over the UK, but more niche areas such as clinical genetics will only have programmes in a few select areas. The implication of this is that if where you train is the most important factor for you, then you need to bear this in mind when deciding the field in which you'd like to specialise.

Non-training posts

As mentioned earlier, doctors who fail to get into specialist training will be moved into career posts which are entered via an intermediate stage, the fixed-term specialist training appointments (FTSTAs). These are one-year jobs in the specialty of choice, and will train doctors up to the same level as those in the first year of the run-through grade. But since they only last a year, at the end of this period doctors in these positions will have to apply for jobs again – either reapplying for run-through training with the aim of building on the knowledge gained in this year, applying to do another FTSTA so that they will gain a level of experience equivalent to two years in the run-through grade, or applying for a dreaded career post. Career posts need three years' post-registration experience, so you will need to have completed two FTSTAs before you can apply for one.

And that whistle-stop tour is about as much as a medical student or junior doctor needs to know about Modernising Medical Careers! The key area that juniors need to know really well is the Foundation Programme, which is the focus of the rest of this book.

Summary

1   The Foundation Programme will last two years, and the first year remains a pre-registration year.
2   You need to start thinking about career plans early, ideally during medical school . . .
3   . . . But conversely, don't go into the foundation years blinkered. Part of the aim of foundation training is to give you experience in a number of specialties and to try them out as possible career pathways.
4   It's a mistake to narrow your options to just one thing you want to do, because it's possible you won't get a training post in that specialty and will be left disappointed. As you go through both medical school

and the foundation years, try to compile a shortlist of specialties that you like, or focus on broad areas, rather than being specific.

5 The location or specialty of the posts that you do in the foundation years will not have any bearing on your application to run-through training, so don't be afraid to break the mould and do something different.

6 Run-through training will have a fixed length, and successful completion will allow doctors to apply for senior medical appointments.

7 Except for the transition between FY1 and FY2, entry at all stages is competitive, with no guarantee of being appointed.

8 Avoid career posts like the plague.

Chapter 2

Applying to join the Foundation Programme: MDAP and MTAS

Introduction

For most medical students, their first experience of MMC will be applying for an FY1 job in the final year of medical school. Leaving no stone unturned in the quest to revolutionise medical careers, this too has been completely revamped.

In the pre-MMC world, appointing people to PRHO posts was easy enough – if the consultant liked you, you'd get the job. How the consultant formed this opinion of you was completely at their discretion. They might pick you on the basis of the CV you submitted, they might remember you as an especially diligent student when you were attached to their firm, they might recognise your name from the rugby club AGM, or you may just have stuck in their mind as the biggest flirt in your year.

This method of appointment had both advantages and disadvantages. On the plus side it meant consultants were able to construct a team that they wanted to work with – and as we all know, a happy team is a productive team! Consultants would also say that their years of experience meant that they were pretty adept at selecting who they believed would make a good doctor, and knowing who would work best with their firm.

Conversely, critics felt that the system was not transparent enough and that there was too much of an old boys' network in place – the age-old arrangement whereby, for example, the doctor who used to captain the chess club only appoints people who have also held this prestigious title. So, all in all, the MMC people didn't like all this and decided that it had to go. And there was another 'problem' with the old system that they felt needed to change – the scheme made it very difficult for people to get a job in a part of the UK away from the medical school that they attended. Now a lot of people would say this is a good thing. The GMC, for one, says that for continuity of education it is much better for students to stay in the vicinity of their medical school. It gives better access to welfare and support services which are vital in a year as difficult as the PRHO one, it makes it easier for medical schools to keep an eye on doctors who struggled as students and who remain their responsibility, and it is recognised that for all students the familiarity of their surroundings aids development and makes for a better doctor. Unfortunately, despite all the arguments against it, pressure from a vocal minority of students who wanted to move and the possibility that equal opportunity laws were being contravened meant that it was decided local matching had to go, and an open national scheme was developed for placing students. Readers, welcome to MDAP.

If you're in medical school then the chances are that MDAP will be an acronym you have heard of. The now infamous Multi-Deanery Application Process was the MMC attempt to bring job allocation into the twenty-first century. No more interviews, no more CVs, no more human contact or even names. In the MDAP world, you became a number in a high-tech computer system that was to sort the wheat from the chaff, and allocate you a job on the basis of the scored value of your submitted application form.

How did MDAP work?

The aim of MDAP was to decide who would be the best candidate for a post by asking applicants to answer a set of questions related to the qualities that most would agree are necessary in a good doctor. At the forefront of the project was the website, www.newdoctor.org. Candidates had to register with this site and answer the following questions.

1 Give two examples of your academic achievements and the significance of these for you.
2 Give two examples of your non-academic achievements and the significance of these for you.
3 Pick two of the seven principles of the GMC's *Good Medical Practice*, state the principle and illustrate your qualities with respect to these.
4 Identify your educational and personal reasons for applying for your first-ranked Foundation School/Deanery or Programme.
5 Teamwork: give two examples in which you have participated and contributed to the successful working of a team.
6 Leadership: give two examples in which you have demonstrated your leadership abilities.

Each question asked for two examples, and each example could score a maximum of four points (*see* Box 2.1), so the highest possible score was 48. Once this was all out of the way (but without knowing their scores), applicants were asked to rank their top 40 jobs in order of preference. As mentioned earlier, final-year medical students are now eligible to apply

---

Box 2.1: How answers were scored on MDAP

0: No evidence provided, i.e. the candidate didn't write anything!
1: Next to no evidence of the stated achievement.
2: Some evidence was given of how the candidate achieved the quality asked for.
3: Good evidence of achievement.
4: A perfect answer, demonstrating exactly how the desired quality was achieved.

all over the UK, so these jobs could come from any two foundation schools in the country.*

With the deadline passed, the forms were marked and scores calculated by the school you ranked as your first choice (i.e. the one from which your first-choice job came) and you were allocated a job. The system of allocating jobs was about as simple as it gets – the highest score gets the job! If two people with the same score went for the same job, then the person who ranked it higher in their list got it. If two people with the same score ranked the same job equally, then random allocation came into play and a computer decided who would get the job.

The problems of MDAP

MDAP was a mess – an absolute catastrophe on a number of levels. An astonishing 581 medical students across the UK were left jobless at the end of the first phase. London's medical students were especially hard hit, with 254 left jobless, representing 44% of the national total, despite Londoners only making up 20% of the UK's student doctors. There were a number of reasons for this almighty cock-up. Many people blamed their medical schools, citing a lack of careers advice and sessions on how to complete the form. While there may be some truth to this, it is worth pointing out that MDAP was sprung on the medical schools, too. On the whole, they didn't know much more than the applicants! However, it is fair to say that the lack of advice given to applicants resulted in many of the problems, as difficulties were caused by people applying only for the most prestigious jobs in the best teaching hospitals. The issue with this is that these jobs attracted all the best applicants, so people who might have been very good ended up missing all 40 jobs for which they had applied, just because each had been allocated to an excellent candidate. This problem could have been solved if people had put down a few 'safety' choices in their application – jobs seen as less attractive, such as those in district general hospitals. London and Manchester suffered the most from this, with both cities seen as cool places to live, with prestigious hospitals in which to work. Given the lack of information, mistakes by candidates in choosing which jobs they applied for are understandable and acceptable. However, what is not acceptable is that some candidates thought they could get away with not answering some of the questions because they regarded them as 'stupid'. Just writing an answer gave candidates one point, so there really is no excuse for writing nothing.

---

* A foundation school is the board responsible for the training of those emerging from medical school, and they're linked to the medical schools. So the North East Thames Foundation School, for example, is the school responsible for all those working in the jobs that were traditionally associated with Barts and the London School of Medicine and Dentistry.

Not all of the problems were due to a lack of understanding of the system, though. The MDAP team need to take a fair amount of the blame. The mistakes were less to do with the form itself, and more to do with the execution of it all. First of all, they missed almost every deadline that they set. When things did happen, they didn't happen very well. With many applicants predictably leaving it until the last minute to submit their application, the traffic overwhelmed the website and it crashed. Many applicants stayed up all night in an attempt to upload their form. When the allocations were announced (delayed, obviously) this same problem occurred again – too much traffic, system meltdown, unhappy students! As you can imagine, all of this didn't make for a very good public impression of the system, and this view was only compounded when it was discovered that the site was not secure – people could easily enter the 'secure' sections and fiddle with the referee statements and application form answers of any candidate. However, what most infuriated both applicants and medical schools was the announcement of the scores. Applicants who scored less than 20 out of 48 were sent a letter telling them that they fell within the bottom 5% of the country, and would have to take an additional assessment of their clinical competency before they would be allowed to apply for jobs. This was despite the fact that there was no mention of this at the start of the process, which was supposed to be a selection procedure, not an assessment process. An apology was later issued for this letter, and no assessment materialised, but it was a PR disaster and the final nail in the MDAP coffin.

Welcome to MTAS

As a result of all this, MDAP has been unceremoniously dropped. In its place, we have the Medical Training Application Service or MTAS, which should be a fresh start. It's being designed by a new company with experience of setting up the NHS jobs website, and it's being built on a completely new architecture – one that we're assured will be free of the technical errors that plagued MDAP. With it come some big changes, two of which in particular stand out as radically different from MDAP. First, you will no longer be applying for jobs, but will instead be applying to join foundation schools – or as they will now be known, Units of Applications (UoAs). The second big change is that the form will no longer be filled out solely by the applicant. In fact, the majority of it will now be completed by your medical school.

Medical school input

One of the major criticisms levelled at MDAP was that it wasn't academic enough, with only 8 out of a possible 48 marks specifically allocated to academic achievement. This amounts to 17% of the form, which doesn't sound like much but doesn't tell the full story, because in reality every question except the one on non-academic achievement could be answered using academic examples. The flexibility of the form was a real strength of MDAP, but unfortunately it has become a casualty of the backlash against the system.

Medical schools were especially concerned that some of their highest achievers were not placed, and MTAS has attempted to solve this problem by allocating a large chunk of marks on the basis of an applicant's academic ranking within their medical school. That's right, all those exams you took under the premise that you only needed to pass will now determine your future career! Goody.

Academic ranking will be worth 45 of the 85 marks available in MTAS, and applicants will be awarded marks according to the quartile into which they fall within their medical school cohort. Did we just hear you ask 'What's a quartile?' Well, in a nutshell, each medical school will rank its final-year students according to their performances in past exams. The exams that can count towards this ranking and the value of each exam will be determined by each medical school at its own discretion. There is no national directive on how medical schools should produce their rankings. The only requirement is that they must be able to show their students how they worked them out. It's at this point that the quartiles come into play. Each ranked cohort will be divided into four groups. The top 25% of a year group will be the highest ranking quartile and will be given a full 45 marks out of 45. Those who make up the next quarter (25–50%) will be the second quartile and will achieve a score of 40 marks out of 45. If you fall into the third quartile you'll be given 35 marks, and if your past exam results put you in the bottom 25% of your year group, you'll score 30 out of a possible 45 marks. It all sounds pretty complex, but in reality it's not too hard to work out. If your year group has 200 students, then those with a ranking of 1–50 will get full marks, those ranked 51–100 will score 40 points, students with a ranking of 101–150 will pick up 35 marks and those with a ranking of 151–200 will score 30 points.

The remaining 40 marks on the form will be filled in by the student as with the MDAP system, but be warned – there'll be an academic question in that part, too! The moral of the story is that you'd best work hard while at medical school or it'll come back to haunt you!

Applying for UoAs instead of jobs

As we've said, with the MDAP system you applied for your 40 favourite jobs in the UK, and these were allocated to the individual who scored highest. This had two major failings. First, it meant that applicants could pick and choose only the best jobs to apply for, which meant that jobs which were deemed prestigious became massively oversubscribed, while less popular ones failed to attract any interest at all. The second problem was that a hospital was bound by the MDAP decision on who to employ, even if they didn't agree with the system's method of deciding what constitutes a good doctor. The MTAS solution to these problems was to change all this and decide that applicants will now apply to join UoAs instead of applying for jobs. Entry to the UoAs will be on the basis of your MTAS score and, as with MDAP, allocation will be on a competitive basis – the higher your score, the greater the chance of getting your first choice. Once you are accepted into a UoA, you're guaranteed a job within it – the question is, which job and how will they allocate them? With MTAS, the responsibility for job allocation has moved from a central system back to the foundation schools. Once MTAS has told each UoA which applicants will be part of their scheme, it is up to them to decide who gets which job. How they make that decision is up to them, and they have three main options available to them.

1   Use the MTAS score and allocate jobs to applicants according to how high they scored.
2   Return to the matching scheme that the foundation school used before MDAP, which could mean CVs, consultant input or interviews.
3   Allocate posts at random.

When it comes to choosing where you apply to, you've got to be realistic and always have a good reason for applying to each UoA. The MTAS site will have a great new feature showing you data on how many jobs each UoA will have, as well as how many people applied for them last year. Use this information wisely and don't apply to just the competitive UoAs. Make sure that there are a few 'easier' options on your list, as it's better to get your tenth choice than to be forced to take a clearing UoA in a part of the country you've never even heard of. Remember, London and Manchester suffered the worst from an excess of applicants, so if you're not a graduate of the medical schools in these areas then have a serious think before you apply to them. The London problem is especially severe. It's the most popular destination for people wanting to leave their home foundation school, but there has always been a chronic job shortage in the capital, with only 800 positions within the M25, despite the fact that London's medical schools produce 1600 graduates a year. The national matching scheme has greatly increased the competition for jobs, so applying to the capital is not something that should be done on a whim!

Making the most of MTAS

So now you know the system, how do you make the most of it? A good start is to familiarise yourself with the website. It sounds obvious, but many of the MDAP generation neglected to do this and only saw the site for the first time when they were uploading their applications. You don't even need to register to browse the MTAS site, so no excuses! Once you do take the plunge and register, you'll have the opportunity to fiddle with your user settings. If you're going on elective during the application period, then the first thing to do is make sure that the email address you're signed up with is fully accessible in the most basic of web browsers. All applicants will automatically be registered with their university email address, but on the whole this isn't the best one to use. Change this to a personal, web-based email account such as Hotmail or Yahoo that you know will load on the 12-year-old PC in a Kenyan DGH! There were no more frustrating problems than those faced by applicants who were abroad during the process and found that they had no way of accessing their application – and this will be especially important for MTAS, as one of the changes this year is that allocation information will now be emailed to you, instead of your only having the option of logging on to the website.

Another common-sense tip is to practise answering the questions online. Take advantage of this because, as mentioned earlier, many applicants to MDAP only tried to log on to the site on the last day, and had problems when it kept crashing. Even though reassurances have been given that this won't happen again, and emailing allocations should ease the pressure, it's still well worth avoiding all the hassle if things do go wrong – so set yourself a strict cut-off point for submitting your application, at least one day before the official deadline. The MTAS site has a very useful feature that enables you to practise answering each question and to save your answer online, so utilise this and you should be fine. It's human nature to want to submit the very best application possible, but if you've been logging on to the site every day to practise your questions, one day won't make much difference! If you're going to be on elective at the time of the deadline, answer the form fully and save your answers before you go.

Summary

1   The infamous MDAP system has been dropped and has been replaced by MTAS.
2   Under MTAS, the application form will be divided into two parts – one section filled in by the medical school and based on an applicant's academic ranking, and the other filled in by the student.
3   Students will now apply to join a UoA instead of applying for individual jobs.
4   Once allocated to a UoA, you are guaranteed a job in it, but the UoAs make their own decisions as to how they will allocate these jobs.

5 Get as much practice on the website as possible, remembering to change your email address to something that you can access on all computers.

6 Practise giving your answers online and don't leave submission of the form until the last minute, however tempting it might be.

7 MTAS will give information on how many applicants a UoA received last year. Use this information and don't apply only to competitive places.

8 If possible, avoid applying to the perennially oversubscribed London UoAs, as it'll all end in tears!

Chapter 3

What makes a good application form?

Introduction

In many ways, this could be taken to mean 'What makes a good doctor?' Indeed, that is what it *should* mean, but everyone realises certain hoops need to be jumped through in order to score highly on your form. However, you should not spend your years at medical school worrying about CVs or application forms. One of the greatest things you can do during your student days is enjoy being a student.

Chapter 4 offers advice for when you come to writing your form, whereas this chapter is concerned with how you can prepare for applying to the Foundation Programme in the preceding years of study. Medical school and university offer a huge range of opportunities, no matter where you study. It would be useless to provide generic advice on how a medical student should spend their free time, but the reality is that as long as you do *something*, writing your form will not be a problem. So what *does* make a good form?

The first myth to dispel is that you need to be a distinction student with a string of academic prizes and publications to your name in order to land a top job. Of course, being top of your class is no bad thing, but don't panic if you have scraped your way through to the fourth year. At present, the emphasis that will be placed on academia for Foundation Programme applications is in a state of flux. Year ranking systems are becoming more popular country-wide, and it is your responsibility to find out whether your medical school will be operating such a system, and if so, how points are allocated. Depending on when you are reading this, you may want to consider directing some efforts towards an academic achievement, but once again – do not fret if your strengths are outside the exam hall.

When thinking about job applications, a few documents deserve a quick glance. Obviously the form itself is key. It may be subject to change from year to year, so make sure that you get your hands on the most up-to-date version. Just as important are the person specification, guidelines for applicants and scorers documents and the GMC's *The New Doctor*, all available via the *New Doctor* website. These will help to guide you as to what you can put on your application, but they make for immensely boring reading, so take a quick look and then put them to one side until you embark upon writing your form.

It is likely that all of the job applications you make throughout your life will place emphasis on some of the same themes – teamwork, leadership and outstanding achievements. However, no matter what questions are asked of you, the beauty of the Foundation Programme application form is that it is eminently flexible. Some students have objected to what they see as a bias in the form, such as an insufficient emphasis on academia. Remember that, for example, academic accomplishments do not have to be limited to the boxes for academic achievements. Participating in a research team during your BSc year qualifies not only as an academic achievement, but also as teamwork, 'maintaining good medical practice' in the *New Doctor* question, or potentially as leadership if applicable. The salient message is that you should not design your student life around your job application form, but design your job application form answers around your student life.

Clichéd though it may be, enjoyment is paramount. If you embark upon a pursuit with the sole motive of having something to put on your form, you are unlikely to enjoy it and hence are unlikely to gain much from it. Frankly speaking, if *nothing* has piqued your interest at medical school, you probably should not expect a stand-out form. Do not despair if this is the case – it is never too late to augment your CV, and mediocre achievements can become admirable with some intelligent writing.

Bearing in mind the answers that you will need to provide on your application to the Foundation Programme, what kinds of things will you need to do in order to cover your bases? The personal statement is your chance to establish that you are in possession of the 'desirable' qualities as specified on the Foundation Programme person specification. A good time to start thinking about what you can say to sell yourself on the job market is around two years before you will be applying for your first house job. For most medical students this will be at the start of the third year in a five-year course. Two thoughts should be at the forefront of your mind. The first you will have heard countless times – that 'rounded personalities' are very much looked for, especially as the Foundation Programme form allows ample opportunity to mention a wide range of extracurricular activities. The second fact is that commitment is held in higher regard than obvious attempts to accrue meaningless titles or positions. Two years or more of concerted effort towards anything like a charity, society or team will sound more impressive than reeling off a list of positions held for merely a few months. Once again, remember that for each answer you give, you are required to reflect upon your achievement, and this is easier if you have actually done something, as opposed to just being vice-deputy co-treasurer of the underwater basket-weaving union.

Academic achievements

This question stipulates that at least one of the answers should be from your time as a medical undergraduate. In fact, unless you are a mature student, it is preferable for both examples of your academic prowess to be from medical school. The exceptions to this would be truly outstanding achievements prior to becoming a medical student, perhaps during school or a previous degree. However, these will be at least five years ago in most cases, so stay contemporary if you can.

In a year group of 300 students, for example, only a handful can boast consistent distinctions or winning top-of-the-year prizes. If you are not one of those brainy few and there is absolutely nothing unique about your exam scores to date, this should not bother you in the slightest. Most people in the year will be just the same. The key to a great personal statement is reflecting on what any achievement meant to you. This means explaining the context, significance and impact of whatever you choose to write about. If you are genuinely proud of simply passing your fourth-year exams while looking after a sick loved one or captaining the athletics team, feel free to say so. The scale of academic feat is not considered in isolation, so demonstrate *why* you chose both of your examples.

Exam prizes come with hard graft. An academic prize looks nice, but it is not the be-all and end-all. With the Foundation Programme form you can mention individual test results, so if you put a bit of elbow grease in for a term and get a spectacular score, that's given you something to write about without needing to work all year round. Perfect for the moderately lazy. Another ideal opportunity for those who might be an intellectual giant in one area of medicine and somewhat of a slouch elsewhere is an optional-entry prize. Obtain a list from your medical school and make sure that you find out what the prizes themselves are. If the ophthalmology prize is £20 in book tokens and the anaesthetics prize is £200 cash, you know which one will be harder to win and you know which one to work for if you are running low on money. The majority of medical schools run at least half a dozen specialty prizes, which normally consist of a brief exam taken during your spare time.

Most medical schools also now include special study modules (SSMs) as part of the course. These represent great opportunities to pursue some-thing in which you are interested. The more engrossed you are in a subject, the better you will do, so treat SSMs as personal projects to excel in. You can work for a good mark, but you could also consider converting an SSM into a spare-time interest and a first-class academic achievement box entry.

For example, suppose that you complete your SSM in the history of pioneering female surgeons and receive a good pass. In a few hours, you have knocked up an article to submit to a medical publication – there are plenty to try. You approach the Surgery Society and you wind up giving an evening presentation. With a bare minimum of additional work, you have a great deal to write about now. This example uses a rather non-academic SSM subject, but exactly the same goes for an SSM on phylogeography of Y-chromosomal lineages in Norway.

A BSc, if you do one, is essentially a jumbo SSM. In fact, if your medical school imposes a limit on the number of students who can undertake a BSc, then being allowed to study for one is an achievement in itself. Treat your project as a chance to get a publication, so pester your supervisor and offer to do the legwork. But more important than anything, do *not* fret if no publications come out of your BSc. Publications come in all guises. Gone are the days when only a paper in the scientific press merited a publication worth mentioning. The Foundation Programme application's looser questions mean that you are the person responsible for making a publication sound impressive. If you are not in a position to do any original research, you will still be able to write academic articles for a host of journals or newspapers.

If one just considers the student press, you should try your university or medical school rag, any of the numerous online medical and medical student websites, or publications like *Medical Student Newspaper* or *student BMJ*. Try pitching an article about an area of interest to you to the editor. For example, a three-part series on cancer treatment in your student paper is far better than nothing. If you get involved with any of these or write a non-academic article anywhere, you will have something for other sections of the application form as well.

Other potential goals to aim for are extracurricular academic prizes. These normally take the form of essay competitions, but can also involve presentations or multimedia. Again, some spare time will have to be sacrificed, but often far less than you think. Your registry will be able to provide you with a list of prizes offered nationally and within your medical school. The Royal Colleges, the BMA and the Royal Society of Medicine all run student competitions, and many have cash prizes or vouchers that you can use for an elective. Research what is on offer, decide your best shot and *have a go*. Fewer people enter than you think, and you could end up with an impressive prize to your name and some money in the bank. You could even be cheeky and repackage that SSM, but unless you try you will not win.

Non-academic achievements

This should be one of the easiest sections, as those who first react by saying 'I have nothing to write' are almost always wrong. Anyone will be able to find two examples to write, and this is the reason why you should try hard to impress here. Some students will take pleasure from academic pursuits, but most will not. Therefore if you fall into the latter category, here is your chance to shine. Non-academic achievements can be anything at all, and as such you are able to choose something you love and pursue it.

Medical school can be tough, and you are expected to spend the majority of every week studying, often with minimal time off. Working as a doctor will be the same. This part of the form is designed to examine your 'work–life balance'. Having an outlet away from work is of vital importance, so taking up a sport, pastime or activity will be of use to you as well as providing something to write about on your form.

As mentioned earlier, commitment garners points, so try to persevere with something you like. It could be playing on the cricket team or performing on stage, writing for a newspaper or DJ-ing for a club full of people. Anything to show you are more than just a head buried in a book. Do not be afraid to mention something unconventional – this is actually more likely to count in your favour. If you are national capoeira champion or you won the Lammy flower-arranging tournament, the examiner does not need to have any specific prior knowledge – you simply have to explain what it is in a few words and indicate your level of proficiency. Marks are awarded for the scale of achievement and diversity, so if you have more than two things to write, try to choose an impressive pair that cover different ground.

Charity work is looked upon very favourably, and if you can show either a lasting dedication to a charity or a single exceptional voluntary action, such as spending a summer working in a developing country, you will be in a great position.

At all times it is essential to be honest, as markers have astute bullshit-detectors. Of course you should not lie at any stage in your job application – you could wind up jobless and facing disciplinary action – but those reading application forms know that students exaggerate and that it often occurs in this section. Make sure you do not push exaggeration too far and think carefully, as you might not need to embellish your activities. The crucial messages to convey are that you are motivated and enthusiastic – what you write about is entirely up to you.

The *New Doctor* principles

This somewhat unusual question was deliberately included to ensure that all candidates read *The New Doctor*. As it currently stands, this section asks you to choose how you embody two of the seven principles of Good Medical Practice as laid out in *The New Doctor* guidelines, published by the GMC. For this reason, the answers in these two boxes will vary widely between applicants. The strategy here is to interpret the principle however you like, so long as you can justify the example that you provide. You can therefore treat this question as a place to mention something you could not put elsewhere, either because it was not appropriate or because space did not permit.

Reflection crops up once again, and in this case it is more integral to your answer than in other sections of the form. Because most of the principles are vague, the validity of your example will depend on your explanation of why it is relevant. This is examined more closely in the next chapter. The *New Doctor* question need not be one that you worry about while at medical school, partly because it may change, but primarily because preparing for the other questions will give you suitable material for this one.

'Good clinical care' is so vague that it is probably advisable to steer clear unless you can put forward a response which you think will fit. 'Maintaining medical practice' essentially means that central to a doctor's career is staying up to date with the latest developments in evidence-based medicine and making sure that their skills remain sharp. The markers are looking for ways in which you demonstrate that you stay abreast of medical matters, but unless this is something significantly more substantial than 'I read the *BMJ*', this may sound a bit woolly. 'Probity' and 'Health' are also probably best avoided. You could potentially cite your daily five-mile run as maintaining your health, but it would be extremely hard to acquire many points with this answer.

'Relationships with patients', 'working with colleagues' and 'teaching and training' are easy boxes to fill. Take 'patients' to read 'the public'. Evidence of your communication skills is being sought. Any activity in which you participate that involves interaction with the public can qualify for an answer, but voluntary work with children, the disabled, the elderly, and so on would be ideal, as it shows that you go out of your way to help members of the public who may well be your patients in the future. 'Working with colleagues' translates as teamwork. Be careful not to duplicate what you will be writing later in the form, under 'teamwork', but if you have more than two examples, use this opportunity. You can demonstrate variety one of your examples of teamwork could be academic and the other two more light-hearted, like writing a rag-week comedy act or organising the summer ball. If you feel that you went out of your way to assist a patient by working as part of a multi-disciplinary team, you can mention this for either of these options. Lastly, 'teaching and training' is best demonstrated by evidence that you impart your knowledge to others. Teaching clinical skills to junior years is a superb way to improve your own technique and to rack up points on your application form. You could tutor your neighbour for their GCSEs, teach as part of a religious group or act as a mentor for schoolchildren wishing to get into medicine, if your medical school runs such a scheme.

Educational and personal reasons

The section concerning educational and personal reasons for applying to your first-ranked Foundation School or Deanery is often the hardest to complete. The overwhelming majority of applicants understandably wish to remain in the area in which they have studied. These questions are liable to change as greater emphasis may be placed upon allowing applicants to work in a hospital allied to their medical school if they so desire. However, somewhat unfortunately, these are two questions where most people will sound very similar. The section is included so that individuals with genuinely pressing reasons for applying to a specific area are given preference. What qualifies as a genuinely pressing reason is open to debate. Although many people simply want to work near their family and friends, this may not score highly on its own, perhaps unfairly.

Educational reasons can potentially be supplemented, for the motivated few. Bear in mind that if you do have something unique to write here, you will almost certainly stand out. Such examples would be ongoing research interests at your medical school, a major audit in which you are participating, or any kind of academic pursuit that would require you to remain close by. Of fundamental importance is explaining your answer, as will be discussed in the next chapter. The vast majority of people will write the same sort of thing, so phrase it well.

Personal reasons are obviously going to be eminently different between applicants. The same applies as for the previous question – any pursuit or responsibility that you will not be able to continue in another location is something to write down. The small proportion of individuals who apply away from their medical school normally do so for a specific reason, so should have no trouble thinking of a reason. Do not lie, and also do not be afraid to be honest. For example, if you feel that you want to stay close to your grandparents, say so. For both sections of this question, read the guidance notes carefully.

Teamwork and leadership

The teamwork and leadership questions complete the form. Providing two examples of each is not necessarily an easy task, so spend your time inside and outside medical school constructively. This does not mean that you cannot lead a normal life – a part-time job could qualify as either leadership or teamwork. Teamwork and leadership can be applied to almost any activity that you decide to pursue, but once again points will be determined by the way that you justify your answers.

Summary

1   You should really start thinking about achievements for your application by your third year but don't design your life around it – do things you enjoy and work out how to include these things in your application form later!
2   Commitment to an activity is far more impressive than doing things for the sake of your CV – put in some long-term work with a charity or a meaningful society.
3   Everyone has some academic achievements they're proud of: SSMs, individual test scores or optional-entry prizes can all be mentioned.
4   Don't even think about lying, ever.

Chapter 4

How to write your application form

Introduction

You're in your final year, within striking distance of putting those two letters in front of your name. All that is left is your application to the Foundation Programme and the small matter of finals. The way that you phrase your answers and the support that you provide for each answer is just as important as what you decide to write about. No points are guaranteed, so spend as much time as you can afford on your form. Exceptional achievements can receive mediocre scores if written poorly and, conversely, quite mundane accomplishments can make a good form.

A sensible way to write your form is to sit down, perhaps with a copy of your CV if you have one, and to list as many achievements as you can. Start in chronological order – before your degree, pre-clinical years, clinical years, and so on. Recall test or examination results and look up coursework grades. Think of as much as you can, and don't limit yourself to activities related to medical school. Make sure that you include jobs you have held, qualifications you have obtained, classes you have taken (e.g. jazz dance, yoga, violin, etc.). Once you are satisfied that you have remembered every possible thing you could be proud of, try to categorise each item on your list. Your categories are dictated by the form – academic, non-academic, the seven *New Doctor* principles, educational and personal reasons for applying to your first-choice deanery, teamwork and leadership.

A prize for the best geriatrics presentation or being selected for a BSc are both obviously academic, but much of what you have done could fit into more than one section. List all of the categories, as you are likely to be chopping and changing your form many times as you construct it. For example, drawing on an elective in which you were given responsibility for patients is a superlative choice. It could qualify for 'working with colleagues', teamwork, leadership and potentially 'relationships with patients'. So now you have a list of your achievements with at least one category beside each of them. Decide which items you definitely want to mention and which you would quite like to. If you are having trouble choosing between more than one entry for a particular box, write answers for them all and assess which one sounds best. Occasionally a slightly less impressive achievement will be more conducive to reflection, so it will actually receive a higher score. It is also worth trying to sound like that magical 'rounded person', so if you find that most of your answers are very serious pursuits, perhaps you could use one of the boxes for a more frivolous activity.

When you have finally decided which 12 answers sound the best, keep reviewing them again and again. Trim them down or pad them out to conform to the 75-word limit. If you are a few words over, be creative with your editing. Shuffle sentences around, hyphenated words count as one word, 'medschool' is a perfectly tolerable alternative to 'medical school', and so on. The word limit is short enough for you to be in little danger of waffling, so don't be afraid to write what you feel.

Academic achievements

The key points can be summarised as follows.

- Anything that shows you are not thick is fair game for inclusion.
- Explain why *you* think it is an impressive achievement (even if you don't, pretend that you do).
- Give an explanation of the achievement itself.
- Give evidence of working outside the basic undergraduate course (e.g. independent projects, BSc, publications).
- Place emphasis on achievements during your time at medical school (they don't have to be medical).
- Think and reflect. Why will each achievement make you a better doctor?

The people marking your form are not foolish, but it is best to assume that they are for most answers. This effectively means making sure that anyone can understand what you mean. Explain your achievements and avoid acronyms like SSM or ULU, although BSc and PhD are acceptable. If you have won a prize, convey how many people were eligible (not necessarily how many people *entered* – there is a subtle difference), what you had to do and what the prize itself entailed.

For any example, try to find a way that it will be relevant to your career as a doctor – this is fundamental. This is normally not difficult for academic achievements, but make an effort to go beyond the obvious. For example, anything self-directed (e.g. SSM, BSc project, article for a magazine) is useful, as you can explain that after medical school almost all the learning you do as a doctor will be self-directed.

Example answer 4.1

I have been awarded distinction or merit grades for all my Special Study Modules. I am proud of this as SSMs represented opportunities to pursue independent and self-directed study of a topic that interested me. The majority of learning I will do in my career as a doctor will be self-directed. I now know that I am able to produce high-quality research on a very wide range of topics and, crucially, to explain it clearly.

The achievement here is laudable but not extraordinary. If you complete five SSMs and one is a distinction and four are given a merit, phrasing your answer like this is economical with words. Admittedly some ambiguity is left, and it is up to your discretion whether you wish to do this, but the answer clearly demonstrates that all of your marks have been above simply a pass. This answer can be tweaked if you excelled in one SSM but fared less well in others – simply talk about that one.

Here you can see a good format – the achievement is explained very briefly and the remainder of the entry is explaining why the examiner should be giving you a 3 or 4. It's also bang on 75 words, and you should always try to use your entire allowance.

BScs are not compulsory at most medical schools, so don't make the mistake of neglecting to mention it somewhere on the form simply because your medical school or university makes it compulsory. At the time of printing, the entire application form does not contain another section in which to mention a BSc. Using one of the academic boxes to talk about your BSc is convenient to most of those who have undertaken an intercalated or previous degree, as it is a significant academic achievement, but if you find that you have several academic feats under your belt on top of a BSc, you might be forced to leave some out, as not mentioning your BSc would be inadvisable.

Even if you already have a doctorate, there are no sure-fire marks in the bag. Hence, for any degree or qualification you must expand upon it.

Example answer 4.2

I was selected to undertake an intercalated Basic Medical Sciences BSc, for which I was awarded a 2.1 (Hons). A limited number of students are allowed to apply for a BSc at St George's, University of London. I combined a genetics research project and physiology module with a special-interest diving medicine module. This BSc gave me experience of designing and completing a laboratory-based research project, as well as studying outside the core medical curriculum.

This is a reasonable answer for someone who has done an average BSc. A first-class or upper-second degree will probably get a higher mark than a lower second or third, and there is little one can change about that. If you have a Desmond (2.2), then writing 'second-class honours' is fine. If you prefer, writing about something specific in your degree is also a good move. Perhaps you entered medicine from a non-scientific background via a graduate-entry degree. In this case, how will your previous degree make you a better FY1 doctor? Consider the non-medical aspects of the job – talking to patients, expressing yourself clearly, dedication, long hours, independent study and more (although try not to mention the same themes in both answers).

Example answer 4.3

During my intercalated Neurology BSc, I particularly enjoyed my research into uncommon neurological diseases. I spent time extensively exploring the rare alien hand syndrome, and decided to write a review article, which was published in the Australian Journal of Neurology. *I also won my university's neurology essay prize. These experiences taught me the skill of collating information from many sources and presenting it succinctly, much akin to explaining a disease or procedure to a patient.*

The last sentence may sound a bit trite, but it will stand your answer in good stead. Here the prize was given a brief mention, as the main achievements are the publication and the BSc, but this answer could ostensibly be divided into two.

One of the best academic achievements will always be getting a distinction or excellent grade for an entire year. A merit is also very praiseworthy, and if you receive any of these for more than just one year you will stand out, as relatively few candidates maintain a high level of performance across the years at medical school. There is plenty to write for the reflection aspect when presenting good examination results.

Example answer 4.4

I gained a 'merit' for both of the first two years, meaning I have been awarded a 'merit' for Stage 1, our pre-clinical years. Only the top 20% are awarded merits, from a year of 250. This reflects my underlying fascination with the subject matter and dedication to study. Pre-clinical years form the basics for every medical field, so thorough knowledge and solid grounding have helped me establish good clinical practice and understand disease processes.

The take-home message is hopefully clear – you will be sick of it by the end of this application form but every answer must be expanded upon. Points are picked up by the way in which you *tell* the marker that your achievement is just what they should be looking for.

Non-academic achievements

The key points can be summarised as follows.

- Give evidence that you are not one-dimensional. Try to make at least one answer portray you as someone who can function completely away from medicine.
- Show that you are someone who knows how to let off steam. Medicine is a stressful career and they want people who can relax.
- Try to include things that make you stand out.
- Feel free to show off to an obscene degree.

If you are having difficulty deciding whether to put an activity here or in a later section, you might want to consider putting your more impressive achievements here. The academic and non-academic achievement sections will place more emphasis on the scale of your deeds, whereas in the *New Doctor*, teamwork or leadership sections you will want to talk more about the relevance of your answer to the required skills. And although there is no guarantee, if one person marks your entire form he or she will be likely to tackle its contents in order, so put your best stuff up front.

Each person is likely to have a different pair of answers for this, so it would be hard to provide a generic guide. But, as above, concentrate on how the activity *has* helped and *will* help you. An overlooked advantage of any non-academic pursuit is that it helps you relax and takes your mind off medicine, which is in fact one of the main benefits, so you may consider mentioning it.

Example answer 4.5

In 2006 I won University Colours, presented for an exceptional contribution to university life. There were only two medical student winners, and the award was open to all 16,000 students at Bristol. I was awarded for 'outstanding service to students' due to being elected third-year rep and a member of the Medical Society. I value this award as I feel proud to have worked to serve my fellow students, particularly organising extra revision lectures.

The achievement comes first, then the background to it, the reason why you were recognised, and finally why you are suggesting this answer. In this case the third-year rep position has not been expanded on too much so that it can be used in another section – thus only the most important aspect has been mentioned. The 'two medical student winners' is an example of a selective revelation. There may have been 30 winners, but this sounds less impressive, so you could highlight the fact that only one other medic was decorated, thereby making your achievement sound better.

Example answer 4.6

I have played the piano since a young age and still enjoy playing regularly. I play keyboard in a band, and we have performed at university, local venues and charity events, including an appearance on BBC Digital Radio. Music allows me to take my mind off work, and I enjoy using my creative side. My band has helped raise money for charity, and I have also been able to supplement my income through modest sales.

Music fits well in here, as it would not be as appropriate in any of the other sections. 'Performing at university' may mean band night in the bar, 'local venues' may mean the pub, 'charity events' may mean a rag-week dinner, 'modest sales' may mean mum, auntie and uncle Jim buying your album, and 'BBC Digital Radio' may mean the BBC Asian Network, but so long as you do not lie, you have nothing to worry about. Make your enjoyment clear, and explain the fact that you like getting away from medicine – it will not be looked upon negatively.

Example answer 4.7

A great passion outside medicine is writing. I regularly write for my student newspaper and an online web log. I cover a diverse range of topics and have had work published in Medical Student Newspaper *and* The Guardian. *I recently won the Malawana Essay Award for an article about the Atkins diet and supermodels. An American consumer website runs this award. My writing ensures I stay extremely up to date with medical and general news.*

If you do have anything journalistic to put down, you can either mention how it keeps you up to date, as is done here, or use the line from a previous example answer, about how writing improves communication skills. Change things round as appropriate, and try not to repeat yourself. Remember that 'maintaining good medical practice' in the next section would also be a suitable place for any answer concerning an activity that keeps you abreast of medical news.

The *New Doctor* principles

The key points can be summarised as follows.

- Your examples do not have to be medical for all of the principles.
- How you embody the principle is important.
- Give evidence that you will keep at least the two principles you mention paramount in your mind as you become a doctor.
- Try to work in things that you wish to write on your form which may not fit elsewhere.

Choose which principles you wish to expand on carefully – only your experiences and your imagination need determine your choice. Below are some suggestions of suitable examples for a few of the principles, but do not feel limited to these if you are confident of giving a solid answer for another. For example, 'good clinical care' is a bit vague for most, but if you have performed an audit on an aspect of clinical care by speaking to patients, this would be ideal.

Do not forget to state which principle you are going to write about, as you might otherwise score zero.

Example answer 4.8

Maintaining good medical practice: I designed and maintain the student union's website. The website is used by a large proportion of the student body. This has meant that my computer proficiency is constantly improving, which is likely to be a valuable skill as a doctor. As I also update the 'latest news' section, I am aware of all the issues that affect medical students, such as changes to training and introduction of the Foundation Programme.

Any mention of computer literacy, provided that you add the line about it being useful for a medical career, will be looked upon favourably, as markers will probably think it is awfully forward-thinking and 2.0 of you.

Example answer 4.9

Working with colleagues: I spent two months volunteering for several hours a day at a home for elderly people with terminal disease. I worked with many inspirational staff members, including nurses, counsellors, pharmacists, dietitians and doctors. As a student I was called upon to help different people, whenever needed. I learned an immense amount about the work involved in a multi-disciplinary team, and realised how important synergy is to providing the best possible care.

This is good, as these other staff members will be your colleagues in the future. Although your interaction with some professions might be minimal when you are a doctor, markers will love to read the 'multi-disciplinary team' buzzword. Doctors can be seen as arrogant, and this attitude often begins at medical school, so show that you are aware that other members of staff are just as valuable as doctors.

Example answer 4.10

Teaching and training: I enjoy teaching colleagues and the public about medicine. I am a clinical skills tutor at medschool and I teach junior students examination techniques. I also produced an information leaflet about diabetes for patients, as part of a Special Study Module. These have taught me that it is vital to tailor information to the audience every time, ensuring the facts are clear and concise. I wish to continue teaching throughout my career.

Make it evident that you will wish to impart the valuable knowledge you pick up not only to patients, but also to other doctors and medical students. Another example you could present is how you explained a complicated condition to a patient and/or their family. Saying that you specifically want to *continue* teaching is excellent.

Educational reasons for applying to your Foundation School

Those of you who have something specific to write here will be at a distinct advantage, but for the average student the following answer will cover most bases. Expressing a desire to stay in the area for years to come can only help. Make sure that you get the name of where you are applying correct. Is it a Foundation School, a Unit of Application or a Deanery? Acronyms for this would be acceptable.

Example answer 4.11

I have enjoyed firms at SWTUoA hospitals immensely, and would very much like to continue the working and academic relationships that I've built up so far. The positions to which I am applying represent hospitals where I met inspirational doctors who have been integral to shaping my interests in medicine. I would very much like to continue to work in this UoA, which has an ethos and patient population I understand well, for many years.

Personal reasons for applying to your Foundation School

Again, this is a section where you either have something to write or you do not. An example answer will probably be unhelpful, as personal situations vary widely from one person to another. The first example is an entry for a typical student with seemingly little to write, and the second is an example of how you can phrase an answer when there is a pressing reason for applying to a certain area. Note that many medical schools have a facility whereby you will be able to ask for special consideration if you have exceptional personal reasons to be taken into account, so enquire if you think that this is something you will need.

Example answer 4.12

I am very family oriented and would like to remain close to my family. I visit them regularly while at university, and would like to maintain my proximity as I begin my working life. I have an established social structure in the Manchester area and my friends and family are very important to me. I would also like to remain close to my medical school to continue friendships with and seek guidance from staff members.

Example answer 4.13

I have lived near my parents throughout medical school as I help them care for my younger sister. She has severe learning disabilities and requires 24-hour care.

My parents are finding it harder to cope without my help as they get older. I am only applying to hospitals near home, which falls in the North West Thames area. During my course, distant attachments have proved very difficult and involved a great deal of travelling.

Teamwork

The key points can be summarised as follows.

- Show that you can work with others while keeping your eye on the final goal or outcome.
- Here the scale of the accomplishment is less important.
- Demonstrate that you know your place in a team – put the wishes of the group ahead of your own.
- Show that you understand the concept of synergy.
- It will do no harm to show that you are even more rounded than they already thought.
- Considering the opinions of others is a useful quality.

Example answer 4.14

I was elected BMA Medical Students' Committee representative for Bart's for the 2005/06 year. This involved voicing views of students at a national level as well as joint projects, in which collaboration was imperative. We delegated jobs, gathered information on our own schools and we worked well together to achieve a great deal. I realised the importance of listening to the views of my colleagues. I learnt how to coordinate efforts towards a common goal.

    If any position you have held is elected, say so. This holds more cachet than other positions. Explain whatever example you choose thoroughly and emphasise the teamwork elements, including any sacrifices you have made and occasions when you have valued and utilised the views of others.

Example answer 4.15

I am a keen dancer and have helped organise and performed in several fashion shows, raising money for RAG. Some of medschool's most enjoyable times have been working with others to produce a great end-product. I have assisted in coordinating rehearsals, choreography and seeking sponsorship. We often filled in for one another to ensure deadlines were met and setbacks avoided. This less formal setting taught me teamwork in a close-knit group and provided much-needed fun.

Example answer 4.16

As entertainments officer for my university, I have been involved with organising many events. Planning and running a large party requires consultation and interaction with bar staff and officers, the president and vice-president, the local police, security services, DJs and often corporate sponsors. It's a hectic process with a very fast turnaround time, but I keep a cool head and we have always managed to run on time and ensure students enjoy themselves thoroughly!

Sports are an obvious choice for teamwork. Even solo sports like squash or athletics tend to be contended between teams. Try to anecdotally explain your teamworking skills if you can recall a suitable incident. If there was an occasion when you went beyond the call of duty to help the group pull through, perhaps you can mention it. Whether it involved staying up all night painting the set for the university play, or playing the last 10 minutes of your netball match with a sprained ankle in order to win the Cup, it may be worth writing about. However, use your discretion to avoid sounding too clichéd and saccharine.

Leadership

The key points can be summarised as follows.

- Leadership entails similar qualities to teamwork, but here the ability to shoulder responsibility is important.
- Show that you have the ability to make decisions.
- Give evidence of others relying on you if possible.
- Providing advice or guidance to others can also be construed as leadership.
- The scale of achievement is not vital here.

Example answer 4.17

I am Deputy Chair of the Surgical Society. The chairman and I are responsible for attracting guest speakers to impart their knowledge to our members. I have also spoken several times at the society's meetings, suggesting ways that medical students can prepare for a career in surgery. I arrange committee meetings and take minutes. I also ensure society evenings run smoothly. Summarising information and organisational competence are key transferable skills for an FY1 doctor.

Example answer 4.18

I captain the university's football 3rd XI. Representing my university and my medical school has given me some of my most enjoyable and proud moments.

Captaining a team requires a calm disposition and the ability to make decisions quickly, by weighing up the relevant variables. I will be doing these things regularly as a doctor. I am used to others depending on me to do my job, and I am happy to take on responsibility.

This is a generic blueprint for any position of responsibility, whether it be in a nursery school or a corner shop. Look beyond the obvious for ways to link what you are writing about to the medical profession.

Example answer 4.19

I am currently the medical school's welfare officer. This position involves guaranteeing the well-being and safety of medical students. I have recently led a policy change in the light of bullying allegations. Two students came to me complaining they had been unfairly treated, and I worked hard to make sure those responsible were disciplined. I will respect the wishes of my patients the same way I stand up for my colleagues' wishes at present.

Example answer 4.20

I spent my elective working in a rural hospital in Siberia. Critical staff shortages meant I was given a great deal of responsibility – I would clerk in, diagnose, treat and discharge patients. I worked closely with other members of staff, and my organisational abilities improved immensely, but the most important transferable skill I learned was that I know when I am out of my depth and when I should ask for senior help.

Summary

1 Start by listing everything noteworthy you have done since your GCSEs, then choose the 12 achievements that fit best.
2 You *will* have enough to write, even if you have spent your medical school years on the sofa watching *Diagnosis Murder*. Think hard.
3 For every section, explain your achievement and then demonstrate why it makes you a good person and a good doctor.
4 Use your word limit in its entirety.
5 Check it, check it and check it again.

Chapter 5

FY1 and starting out as a doctor

What it's all about

The Foundation Programme was introduced by Modernising Medical Careers (MMC) in response to concerns which arose from an evaluation of the previous Senior House Officer (SHO) grade. The lack of an explicit curriculum, combined with inadequate supervision and progression linked to time served and not competences achieved, had led to the evolution of an ill-defined system of subjective assessment and advancement in the early years after graduation.

Enter the Foundation Programme. This ambitious initiative sets out a nationally approved framework for the continuing education of newly qualified doctors. In doing so, it aims to provide medical graduates with much needed guidance and remove a significant proportion of ambiguity from the previously murky waters of postgraduate education, as well as providing continuity from medical school through to specialist training. Put simply, it is a bridge from one to the other.

This overhaul in postgraduate medical education is a world first, and represents just one of a series of changes to the same being devised as part of MMC. An overhaul of specialty training is also in the pipeline and will be in place in August 2007.

To accompany these drastic reforms, a large amount of literature has been produced on the subject of the Foundation Programme. Much of this is beyond the scope of these chapters, whose purpose is to flesh out the basic details of the foundation years which students may already have come across, without overwhelming the unwitting reader with unnecessary detail. We hope that you find this information useful.

How the Foundation Programme works

All UK medical graduates are now required to undertake the Foundation Programme before progressing to specialty or GP training. Doctors with a medical degree gained outside the UK who are eligible for provisional registration with the General Medical Council (GMC) will also be required to complete the programme.

In the final year of medical school, doctors-to-be will apply for their first job, and consequently a place at a foundation school. Currently any student can apply to anywhere in the country. The selection process is based on fair and open competition between both UK students and overseas graduates.

Assuming that the offer of a job is made, and finals are passed, new doctors will gain provisional registration with the GMC upon graduation (*see* Box 5.1), and will enter Foundation Year 1 (FY1) in August of the same year. This year is equivalent to the old pre-registration house officer (PRHO) year, and doctors will be given the formal title of 'Foundation House Officer 1'.

Box 5.1: Provisional GMC registration[1]

1 The GMC visits students at every medical school in either the fourth or final year in order to verify the identity of applicants for provisional registration.
2 Following this check, a GMC reference number, PIN code and password will be sent to you to enable you to access the secure area of the GMC website, MyGMC.
3 On receipt of your degree certificate, go to www.gmc-uk.org and log into MyGMC. Check that your details are correct.
4 Pay the fee for provisional registration (currently £100). This can be paid online.
5 Your registration will automatically be activated. You don't need to send your degree certificate to the GMC, as all universities supply the GMC with a list of successful candidates. You will be sent a certificate to confirm your provisional registration.

Note: You *must* be provisionally registered before you begin work in FY1. Work while unregistered is not legally covered and may invalidate all or part of your FY1 experience. Don't assume that you have been registered until you are looking at the certificate. It pays to give a secure address!

On satisfactory completion of FY1, doctors will be eligible for full registration with the GMC. They will then enter Foundation Year 2 (FY2), which replaces the first year of traditional senior house officer (SHO1) training. During FY2, trainees will have the opportunity to sample a variety of specialties. The title of 'Foundation House Officer 2' will be given to doctors at this stage.

Throughout the Foundation Programme, doctors will be assessed against a list of explicit competences detailed in the *Curriculum for the Foundation Years in Postgraduate Education and Training* (the *Curriculum*).[2] This document was agreed upon by the GMC and the Postgraduate Medical Education and Training Board (PMETB) – the bodies which assume overall responsibility and quality assurance for FY1 and FY2, respectively.

After finishing the Foundation Programme, doctors will receive a Foundation Achievement of Competency Document (FACD), and will be permitted to apply for higher training posts.

Essentially, this reworking of postgraduate training should be beneficial to trainees as well as to their patients. Pilot results have indicated that fewer doctors are undecided in terms of career choice after experiencing a variety of specialties, and the structured training and breadth of experience have been identified as key benefits of the programme.

How the Foundation Programme is organised

All postgraduate training and education is now administered through foundation schools, which consist of all the institutions involved in the training of junior doctors, including trusts, medical schools, the local deanery and other organisations. There are currently 26 foundation schools, each of which accommodates around 300 foundation doctors. Each school is led by a school director and overseen by a postgraduate deanery. A Foundation Programme Training Director (FPTD) is responsible for around 30 trainees, who share a specific foundation training programme.

Information on the roles and responsibilities of the individuals and organisations involved in foundation training is available in the *Operational Framework for Foundation Training* (the *Framework*).[3]

The aims of the programme

The Foundation Programme has been designed around seven specific principles:

1 assessment of competences achieved, not time served
2 service-based structure, aiming to combine clinical care for patients with training for doctors and reinforcing the importance of 'learning on the job'
3 quality assurance, with all doctors produced being competent to serve the general public
4 flexibility of training, with a variety of different learning opportunities available
5 well-defined structure of the curriculum, with time earmarked for teaching
6 streamlined transition between medical school and specialty training
7 trainee-focused programme that responds to the needs of its candidates.

With these principles in mind, the programme aims to produce doctors who are not only competent in core clinical skills, but have also learned other vital skills for working effectively in the modern NHS, including teamworking, communication skills and the use of evidence and data. Such was the original concept of the Foundation Programme as described in *Unfinished Business*, published by Chief Medical Officer Sir Liam Donaldson in 2002.[4]

As you sift through the paperwork available, it is likely that you will come across numerous other goals, principles, aims and foci of the Foundation Programme. You will discover that the programme is structured, streamlined, standardised, homogenised and pasteurised. It is also service based, workplace based and competence based, as well as trainee centred, assessment centred and, of course, patient centred!

The message is that the Foundation Programme has numerous aims and ideals, many of which are worthy and should be striven for, but the volume (and buzzwords) of which tend to cause the bewildered reader to lose sight of the salient points. We believe that these can be identified as the following.

1   The Foundation Programme structures the previously vague period of time between medical school and specialist training.
2   It should produce doctors who are competent to go on to train in any field of medicine – it's for getting the basics right.
3   That's it.

So as we distil the relevant information into these pages, remember that most of the objectives of the Foundation Programme relate to the above!

Getting started as a new doctor

Before starting work

After finishing finals, no doubt boring paperwork will be the last thing you want to face. But there are one or two matters you should take care of before jetting off to the Bahamas.

1   Ensure that you've been provisionally registered with the GMC (*see* Box 5.1).
2   If you didn't do so while in medical school, join a defence body such as the Medical Protection Society or the Medical Defence Union, or take out personal indemnity insurance. The automatic NHS indemnity scheme only covers work done within the NHS – it does not cover work outside the NHS, 'good Samaritan' acts or work overseas. Defence bodies also provide legal advice on matters arising from your work.
3   Ensure that you have received a formal job offer, contract and job description from the trust with which you will be taking up employment.

Contracts and job descriptions

As a new employee of a trust, you will soon have rights and responsibilities in this respect as well as in your role as a doctor. Your contract and job description will underpin many of these, and it is advisable to take time to read both thoroughly.

To begin with, if you haven't received these documents by the time you graduate, you should write to the Human Resources department at the trust and request them. Trusts are obliged by law to provide you with the documents, and normally they are sent to new doctors along with the formal job offer. At the very latest, you must have a job description by the time you have been in a post for two months. There ought to be a separate job description for each placement that you do. Box 5.2 lists what is and is not included in the job description of a PRHO.

Box 5.2: What you should and should not be doing as an FY1 doctor[5]

You should be:
- clerking patients
- taking part in ward rounds
- requesting investigations and chasing results
- performing practical procedures
- doing some administrative tasks, including updating patient lists and theatre lists, writing discharge summaries and completing death certificates
- communicating progress to patients and their relatives.

You should not be:
- delivering requests or samples by hand, or chasing X-rays – secretarial and ward clerk support should be available
- performing day-case endoscopy or angiography, unless this is in the context of your education or in the interests of continuing patient care
- performing exercise ECGs or minor surgery, unless there is a clear element of training for you.

Secondly, you should know that the BMA negotiated standard national contracts and job descriptions for each grade of junior doctor a few years ago, in collaboration with the Departments of Health in the UK. However, this doesn't always prevent trusts from adding their own clauses.[6] You should compare your contract with the relevant model, available via the BMA, and view any additions with a high index of suspicion. The main pitfall to watch out for is any authorisation for deductions from your salary. In the standard contract there is a clause (paragraph 14) prohibiting the trust from making deductions from your salary, other than those required by law, without your express written consent. The deductions required by law are income tax, national insurance and superannuation (plus, of course, student loan repayments). Sometimes trusts will try to leave out this paragraph, or get you to agree to striking out references to it. Alternatively, you might be asked to sign an agreement to salary deductions for phone calls, wear and tear on accommodation, or even a blanket authority for multiple deductions. Do not sign any of these agreements. Box 5.3 lists the dos and don'ts of NHS contracts.

Box 5.3: Dos and don'ts of NHS contracts

Dos
- Do take your time over reading the contract and job description.
- Do contact your local BMA office if you have concerns about either of these.
- Do double-check that paragraph 14 is in your contract.

Don'ts
- Don't sign a contract before you graduate (just in case!).
- Don't sign a letter of acceptance or contract on your first day – take it home and read it first.
- Don't believe that you won't be put on the payroll if you don't sign something on your first day.

The important thing to remember is that once signed, the contract binds not only the trust but also you. Subsequent alterations cannot be made without written mutual agreement, which may be difficult to obtain.

Signing a non-standard contract may prove costly, so it is advisable to check anything you are unsure about with your local BMA office (advice and contract checking require BMA membership). Box 5.4 provides a checklist of the information that should be clear from your contract and job description.

Box 5.4: Information in the standard contract[6]

- Hours and pattern of work (on-call rota, part or full shift, and how many doctors you share this pattern with).
- Salary and job band (i.e. standard working week pay plus a supplement for out-of-hours work, described as a banding).
- Leave entitlement (5 weeks' paid annual leave, divided into 6-month periods; some or all of the leave may be fixed within the rota).
- Arrangements for cover when colleagues are on leave.
- Start and finish dates of your employment.
- Notice of termination you must give or be given.
- Limitations on your obligation to do unpaid work.

The BMA, as the UK doctors' trade union, has published extensive material on the details of NHS contracts and related issues. The *Junior Doctors' Handbook*[7] deals with terms and conditions of service and employment matters, and is an excellent place to start. It is sent free of charge to all junior doctor BMA members and is available through the BMA website.[8] The *studentBMJ* has published several articles summarising the main points about NHS contracts[6] and the problems that might be faced by FY1 doctors,[9] which are available online.

The first day: induction

Induction courses will be held at trusts across the country at the start of the year. This is to familiarise you with the hospital, your timetable and what is expected of you. Expect to receive information on the layout and facilities of the hospital, the bleep system, infection control, local prescribing policies, and test ordering and reporting methods. There will also be a departmental induction for each new placement in the Foundation Programme, in which you will meet your new team.

At the hospital induction, it is likely that you will also be given a small mountain of paperwork and other goodies, including:

1 the details of the administrator to whom you will be expected to give your completed assessment forms
2 the contact details of your named educational supervisor and clinical supervisor
3 the ultimate status symbol – the bleep.

Whereas in 2005, new doctors were provided with backpacks containing important documents about the Foundation Programme, it now seems that you will be expected to download your own copies from the MMC website. These documents include the *Curriculum*,[2] the *Rough Guide to the Foundation Programme* (the *Rough Guide*)[10] and the *Framework*.[3] A *Foundation Learning Portfolio*[11] should also be given to you. Website addresses for these items can be found at the end of this chapter.

Your educational supervisor is the consultant or GP supervisor who will be your first contact in terms of your educational needs. You will discuss your assessments with them, and they will undertake appraisals, review your portfolio, and set educational goals with you at regular intervals. They will also report to the deanery on your progress at the end of the year, hopefully recommending you for full registration with the GMC. It is in your interests to strike up a good relationship with them! In many foundation schools your educational supervisor will be the same for all of FY1, or even the length of the programme, but in some instances they may change with each placement, just to keep you on your toes. Whichever is the case, you should always have access to adequate educational support. They will all have been trained for the role.

The clinical supervisor is the doctor who will oversee your day-to-day clinical work and support your assessments. There will be a different one for each post, but you may find that your educational and clinical supervisors are one and the same person.

Box 5.5 lists the documents that you need to bring on your first day to make it run as smoothly as possible.

You should also aim to get the low-down on other essentials, such as parking facilities, computer access, work rotas, ID badges and access codes, as soon as possible. The *Oxford Handbook for the Foundation Programme*[5] contains comprehensive information on what you should remember to do at the start of your post.

Box 5.5: Paperwork for Day 1[5]

- Latest P45 or P60 form.
- Bank details.
- GMC certificate.
- Criminal Records Bureau (CRB) certificate if you have one.
- Evidence of hepatitis B status (immunity and vaccination record).
- Any documents sent to you by the trust beforehand (e.g. contract).

Accommodation

As an FY1 doctor you will be required to be resident in the hospital when on call, as a condition of your appointment. The trust is therefore obliged to provide you with lodgings, free of charge. If you would rather rent alternative accommodation, the price of this may be reduced by the amount that the offered accommodation would normally cost.

Unfortunately, there is no requirement for trusts to provide FY2 doctors with accommodation. They may be able to advise you about local accommodation, or even have rooms available ('voluntarily resident practitioners'), but there will usually be a charge for this.

Standards of accommodation vary, but basic standards have been agreed upon by the BMA and the Department of Health. Information on this and more can be found in the *Junior Doctors' Handbook*.[7]

Salaries

The salaries for FY1 and FY2 doctors will be the same as they were in the old system for PRHOs and SHOs, respectively. Each grade has its own basic pay scale, with three entry points on the PRHO/FY1 scale, and seven on the SHO/FY2 scale. On appointment to a grade you will normally be paid at the minimum rate for that grade, but once you have experience you should be placed at a higher point on the scale.

Banding (a pay supplement to reflect out-of-hours work and intensity) will still apply to any post that requires an out-of-hours on-call commitment, but not all posts will have this. For example, in general practice, most placements will involve normal working times only. Academic placements will only be eligible for banding if there is an out-of-hours service commitment, which there may well not be.

Foundation schools will seek to ensure that their trainees are allocated a range of posts, so it is likely that some of your posts will be subject to banding, whereas others will not.

All training posts must be monitored for at least 2 weeks every 5 months to check that the banding which they are allocated accurately reflects the hours of the job. Should your post be found to have an incorrect banding, your salary may increase, but it is protected against a decrease.

The *Junior Doctors' Handbook*[7] advises new doctors to contact the previous holder of the post that they are due to take up, in order to check that the arrangements of the post – in particular the banding – have not been surreptitiously altered between employees.

The NHS Careers website[12] contains information on the current pay scales for doctors. Further information on salaries and banding can be sought from the foundation school within your deanery.

Working hours

All foundation posts will comply with the European Working Time Directive (EWTD) (UK law) and the New Deal (an agreement between the UK Departments of Health and the BMA), which together set out rest requirements and weekly working time limits for employees. Effectively, the EWTD means that junior doctors currently cannot work more than 58 hours on average per week. In August 2007 this will be further reduced to 56 hours, and in August 2009 junior doctors should only be working a comfortable 48 hours per week.

The New Deal dictates a maximum of 56 hours of actual work (on your feet) per week, with a total duty of 72 hours a week, including on-calls. You are also entitled to a 30-minute paid break for every 4 hours' continuous work (see the *Junior Doctors' Handbook*[7] for more information on the EWTD and New Deal legislation).

Structure of FY1

The first year of the Foundation Programme is similar to the old PRHO year, in that you must undertake at least 3 months each of both medicine and surgery in order to be eligible for full registration with the GMC at the end of the year. Some rotations will still comprise 6 months of each, but most have changed to offering three 4-month attachments in FY1 (*see* Worked example 5.1).

The placements themselves are determined by the post or programme for which you are selected through the admissions process. These may include any of the 65 recognised specialties in addition to general medicine and surgery. Each foundation school will have a different list of specialties available to its trainees, but all combinations should provide ample opportunities for you to work towards the core competences of the Foundation Programme. Again the emphasis is on getting the basics right.

At the end of each FY1 placement, you will be issued with a 'Certificate of Satisfactory Service'. You will need to send these certificates as you receive them to the nominated person at the university where you graduated. This is to enable them to sign off your 'Certificate of Experience' at the end of FY1, and for you to be recommended for full registration with the GMC.

Worked example 5.1: FY1 placement combinations

James: 6 months acute medicine, 6 months surgery
June: 4 months acute medicine, 4 months surgery, 4 months gynaecology

---

The curriculum in FY1

The content of both years of the Foundation Programme is based on the *Curriculum*,[2] which currently stands to be updated by the Royal Medical Colleges in early 2007, ready for the cohort of new doctors in August of that year.

The *Curriculum*[2] contains both a list of specific competences and a syllabus. The competences – educational objectives of the programme – are grouped into levels of ability for FY1 and FY2, and relate to the GMC's seven principles of *Good Medical Practice (GMP)*.[13] They will form the basis of your assessments as a foundation doctor. Box 5.6 provides an overview of the core competences of the Foundation Programme, as found in the *Curriculum*.[2]

The syllabus describes in detail the core skills, knowledge and attitudes required of a doctor upon completion of the Foundation Programme. Both parts of the document can be used as checklists to guide your training.

Box 5.6: Core competences of the Foundation Programme[1]

1 Good clinical care:
   - practising medicine to a high standard
   - staying within the limits of your ability
   - not putting patients at unnecessary risk.
2 Maintaining good medical practice:
   - keeping up to date with knowledge in your field
   - keeping your clinical and non-clinical skills honed.
3 Partnership with patients:
   - developing and maintaining professional relationships with patients
   - understanding patients' expectations and experience of healthcare.
4 Working with colleagues and in teams:
   - working as an effective team member within the multi-disciplinary team.
5 Assuring and improving the quality of care:
   - understanding clinical governance
   - constantly ensuring that care given is of good quality, safe and appropriate to the needs of patients.
6 Teaching and training:
   - being effective in educating colleagues, patients and their relatives.
7 Probity:
   - being honest at all times.
8 Health:
   - maintaining your own health so as not to put patients, colleagues or the public at risk.

The *Curriculum*[2] is designed to follow the principle of 'spiral' learning, whereby similar subject matter is revisited at increasing levels of complexity and in different situations.

The *Framework*[3] is the companion document to the *Curriculum*,[2] and is the ultimate guide to the way in which the Foundation Programme will be implemented.

Formal teaching in FY1

The professional elements of the *Curriculum*[2] are addressed in a formally taught educational programme, and you will be granted up to 3 hours per week of bleep-free time to attend (or, at some deaneries, 7 whole days of

Table 5.1 Examples of teaching methods that may be used as part of the Foundation Programme

Teaching method	Example
Learning by experience	Ward rounds, supervised consultations
Small group learning	Bedside teaching, group skills training
One-to-one teaching	Case presentations with educational supervisor
External courses	Lectures, formal training
Role models	Emulating senior colleagues, discussion of leadership skills
Simulations	Patient safety drills
Audit	Joint audit project in FY2 with other trainees
Personal study	Personal reflection, background reading

study time every 8 weeks). This study time is arranged by the foundation training programme director (FTPD). There is no study leave in FY1.

A number of recommendations have been made for the delivery of teaching and training within the Foundation Programme, as illustrated in Table 5.1. You should expect to be taught using a range of these methods during FY1.

The topics that will be emphasised in formal teaching during FY1 will include clinical governance and patient safety. You will also be taught about safe prescribing, risk management, legal responsibilities, cultural awareness and organisational skills.

Assessment and feedback

Why?

As the *Rough Guide to the Foundation Programme*[10] explains, the assessment in the Foundation Programme serves several purposes. First, the system must be accountable to the public. That doctors have proved their ability to practise medicine in accordance with the standards set by the GMC is crucial to patients' faith in their healthcare system.

Secondly, assessment and feedback supply you with a method of tracking your progress and achievements over the course of the early years of training. This will help to identify any areas of difficulty so that assistance may be given as soon as possible and in confidence. It will also get you used to continual learning as a matter of course in your career.

Finally, evidence of your performance will influence your educational supervisor's report to the deanery at the end of the year. A good report is imperative to ensure that you are granted full registration with the GMC.

How and where?

The assessments aim to capture what actually goes on in the workplace, so will be incorporated into your everyday practice. This is to allow your educational supervisor to see how you work on a day-to-day basis, and to witness your ability to put into practice the knowledge that you have acquired, rather than your ability to perform in artificial situations.

Methods

There are four newly established 'tools' for the assessment of trainees in the Foundation Programme, each with a catchy abbreviation. You'll be told which of these apply at your foundation school at the start of the programme. You will also be able to collect a timetable indicating deadlines for completion of your assessments from your local deanery.

At the beginning of the Foundation Programme you will receive a pack of assessment forms for three of the assessment tools. These tools will involve you asking more senior health professionals to assess you, and their subsequent completion of a form. After each assessment, it is your responsibility to hand the relevant copies to your Foundation Programme Administrator (FPA) and educational supervisor, while keeping the remaining copy for your portfolio. The fourth tool is a form of peer evaluation, and comes in two varieties, as will be explained later.

The assessments will be based on the foundation competences listed in the *Curriculum*.[2] However, as there are so many, not all of the competences will be examined. You will have to ensure that you have been assessed in each of the groups listed in order for a 'global' assessment to be made at the end of the year. It is important that you do this, as your full registration with the GMC is subject to your satisfactory completion of the FY1 assessments.

Table 5.2 summarises each type of assessment, including the number of each type of assessment required per year, and the estimated time required for each. The tools are described in more detail below.

Direct Observation of Practical Skills (DOPS)

This tool is designed to assess trainees' grasp of specific essential procedural skills. Each assessment focuses on an individual practical skill, and different observers evaluate each of the DOPS assessments that a trainee

Table 5.2 The different assessment tools used in FY1

Tool name	Description	Main skills assessed	Estimated time required	Number in FY1 (minimum)
DOPS	Structured checklist accompanying procedure	Procedural skills	20 minutes	6
Mini-CEX	Assessment of doctor–patient interaction	Clinical skills, professional attitudes and behaviour	20 minutes	6
CbD	Discussion about a case that has been seen	Clinical reasoning/ judgement and patient management	20 minutes	6
MSF: Mini-PAT	Questionnaire completed by co-workers plus self-rating form	Professional attitudes and behaviour	6 minutes × 8 assessors	2
MSF: TAB	Questionnaire completed by co-workers	Professional attitudes and behaviour	3 minutes × 10 assessors	1

undertakes within the year. The observer may be an experienced consultant, Specialist Registrar (SpR), senior SHO (above SHO1), nurse or career-grade doctor in the secondary care setting, or a GP trainer, GP or experienced general practice nurse in the primary care setting.

The procedure itself is selected by the trainee from the list of core problem groups in the *Curriculum*.[2] Examples might include the insertion of a nasogastric tube or cannula, administration of an intravenous infusion, or measurement of an arterial blood gas. It might be suggested that the procedures listed for the DOPS tool are too elementary, but the emphasis of the tool lies in getting the basics right. The assessor indicates on the form whether the procedure is of low, average or high difficulty.

The assessor awards a mark out of 6 for each of the following 11 criteria:

1 understanding of indications, relevant anatomy and technique of procedure
2 obtaining informed consent
3 pre-procedure preparation
4 appropriate analgesia or safe sedation
5 technical ability
6 aseptic technique
7 seeking help where appropriate

8   post-procedure management
9   communication skills
10   consideration of patient/professionalism
11   overall ability to perform procedure.

A score of 4 indicates that the trainee meets expectations for an FY1 or FY2 leaver, according to which year they are currently in. A score of 3 indicates borderline competence, a score below 3 is below expectations for completion of the year and a score above 4 is above expectations. This marking scheme is used for all of the assessment tools.

To gain maximum benefit from this assessment, you should be assessed performing procedures which you do on a regular basis, in the environment in which you normally do them (in other words, not the clinical skills laboratory!).

Mini-Clinical Evaluation Exercise (Mini-CEX)

Originally designed by the American Board of Internal Medicine, the Mini-CEX involves the assessment of a consultation between a patient and the foundation doctor, and evaluates the clinical skills, professional attitudes and behaviours of the trainee.

The assessment focuses on a different clinical problem each time, and trainees will have selected a problem from each of the acute-care scenario groups listed in the *Curriculum*[2] by the end of the year. These are summarised on the assessment form as pain, airway, breathing, circulatory, psychological/behavioural and neurological problems. The focus of the clinical encounter is chosen each time from the categories of history, diagnosis, management and explanation.

The following areas are examined by this tool:

- history taking
- physical examination skills
- communication skills
- clinical judgement
- professionalism
- organisation/efficiency
- overall clinical care.

Not all areas need to be examined on every occasion. Those that are examined are awarded a mark out of 6, where again a score of 4 indicates that the requirements of the foundation year in question have been met.

A different observer should witness each assessment. This may be an experienced consultant, SpR, senior SHO (if they have relevant experience with the case) or career-grade doctor in the secondary care setting, or a GP trainer or GP in the primary care setting. The observer rates the case in question as low, average or high in terms of complexity. More importantly, they provide the foundation doctor with immediate feedback on their performance and will help them to identify their strengths and weaknesses.

Again, the benefit of the assessment is maximised if you do what you do in everyday practice. It is not designed to be a 'long case' assessment with an overly detailed examination, for example.

Case-based Discussion (CbD)

The simple concept of discussing patients with (or presenting them to) more senior colleagues has been transformed into a tool whereby foundation trainees can receive structured assessment and feedback. This goes by the name of 'chart-stimulated recall' in the USA and Canada, and is widely used to assess residents and other doctors encountering problems.

The trainee selects two cases of patients whom they have recently seen and in whose notes they have made entries, and preferably gets them to the assessor before the assessment. The assessor then chooses one of these cases to use for the assessment on a mutually agreed date. The case is classified into one of the clinical problem categories, in a similar fashion to the Mini-CEX, and is also rated as low, average or high in terms of complexity.

The discussion of the case focuses on the foundation doctor's entry in the notes of the patient in question. In doing so, it evaluates the trainee's application of medical knowledge and clinical decision making to the care of their patients. The dialogue may also touch on the legal and ethical aspects of practice, and provides an opportunity for reflection on the particular course of action taken and the possible alternatives.

The precise areas that are examined and marked out of 6 are as follows:

- medical record keeping
- clinical assessment
- investigation and referrals
- treatment
- follow-up and future planning
- professionalism
- overall clinical judgement.

As with the Mini-CEX, a focus of the clinical encounter is selected, this time from medical record keeping, clinical assessment, management and professionalism.

The timing and cases are selected by the trainee. The observer is also selected by the foundation doctor, and may be an experienced consultant, SpR, senior SHO (if they have relevant experience in the case) or career-grade doctor in the secondary care setting, or a GP trainer or GP in the primary care setting. At least one of the CbD assessments in each clinical placement must be with the supervising consultant.

Multi-Source Feedback (MSF)

There are two tools for this type of appraisal – the Mini Peer Assessment Tool (Mini-PAT) and the Team Assessment of Behaviour (TAB). Both tools are used to gather information from a spectrum of co-workers in order to obtain a so-called '360° assessment'. Foundation schools may use one or both of these tools.

Mini-PAT

The Mini-PAT involves the trainee nominating eight assessors to rate them, who may be consultants, GP principals, career-grade doctors, SpRs, SHOs, other foundation doctors and experienced nursing staff or other allied health professionals (AHPs). You are advised to choose people from a range of professions and grades, and with whom you regularly work. If you have been in your current post for less than 3 months, you can choose some or all of your assessors from your previous placement.

To nominate your assessors, you must fill in an 'Assessor Proposal Form' with the names, positions and contact details of your nominees. It is polite to ask your potential assessors' permission first, and to indicate that you would appreciate their feedback.

You must also complete a 'self Mini-PAT', which is the same form as the one that the assessors are given. This and the nomination form should be returned to your Trust Foundation Administrator (TFA). The assessors are then each sent a questionnaire to fill in, and you don't need to do anything more.

The areas for which you and your colleagues are asked to give a score out of 6 are as follows:

- good clinical care (e.g. ability to diagnose patients' problems)
- maintaining good medical practice (e.g. ability to manage time effectively)
- teaching and training, appraising and assessing (e.g. willingness/ effectiveness when teaching or training colleagues)
- relationship with patients (e.g. communication with patients)
- working with colleagues (e.g. ability to recognise and value the contribution of others).

The assessors can also write free-text comments on your progress, and have the opportunity to voice any concerns about your probity or health.

Feedback from your assessors is combined electronically at the assessment centre in Sheffield and is placed online on a secure website to which your administrator will have access, within 6 to 8 weeks of submission. The analysis is presented as a chart illustrating the mean assessor rating, the self-assessed rating and the national mean rating. Free-text comments are included verbatim but are anonymous.

The results are then discussed by the trainee and their educational supervisor, and strengths and areas for improvement are identified from the collated feedback.

Foundation schools that use the Mini-PAT will conform to two national dates for the assessments. These are likely to be in October/November and February/March. A more accurate timeline is available on the Healthcare Assessment & Training website.[14]

TAB

The second form of multi-source feedback, the TAB, is much the same in that the trainee nominates their assessors, but for this tool, 10 assessors are required, and their diversity is more specific. At least five should be qualified nurses, preferably of ward-sister level, and three should be doctors, one of whom should be the current supervising consultant or GP. The remainder may be drawn from the same pool of professionals as the Mini-PAT, with the addition of laboratory staff, therapists and other colleagues.

The trainee will receive and distribute a minimum of 10 TAB forms, which include envelopes addressed to the Foundation Programme Training Director (FPTD). Some programmes will require the trainee to copy the form from their portfolio for their assessors. You need to ensure that a minimum of 10 assessors have completed and returned their forms in order for reliable feedback to be generated. It is in your interests for as many people as possible to fill in the forms so that the reliability of the results reduces their overall subjectivity. In other words, one person's low opinion of you should be brought up by the law of averages. Your assessors are asked to consider your behaviour over time rather than on one or two isolated occasions. They are also discouraged from using the tools as a way of venting a personal dislike, although this cannot always be prevented.

Assessors are asked to indicate whether they have 'no concern', 'some concern' or 'major concern' about the trainee's behaviour in the following areas:

- maintaining trust/professional relationships with patients (e.g. respecting patients' opinions)
- verbal communication skills (e.g. speaking at appropriate levels for patients)
- teamworking/working with colleagues (e.g. working constructively as part of a team)
- accessibility (e.g. taking responsibility and only delegating when appropriate).

Feedback from the assessment is relayed to the trainee via their educational supervisor. Again, all written comments are given word for word, along with a summary sheet showing the ratings given by the assessors, which will be included in the trainee's portfolio.

Any weaknesses that crop up can be addressed at the time of receiving feedback, along with any concern markers. The programme director may wish to discuss any 'major concern' markers with the assessors concerned, and possibly arrange further TAB assessments.

You should also note that since assessors complete MSF forms on the understanding that their confidentiality will not be breached, you will be unable to find out who wrote what in the free comments section. The benefit of this, of course, is that the feedback is more likely to be honest!

In most cases the MSF tools are likely to generate gratifying positive feedback for your portfolio.

Other assessment methods

Despite the apparent rigidity of these assessment tools, there are other ways of proving your salt. As well as reflective pieces, you may want to submit certificates from training courses, project work or even personal references. The *Curriculum*[2] also indicates that assessment of your portfolio, or other tools such as video assessment or critical incident analysis, may be used. You will be told exactly what applies at your foundation school at the start of the programme.

A list of the core competences and suggested tools for each of them can be found in the *Rough Guide*.[10] The total amount of assessment time per trainee is expected to be around 40 minutes per month.

Standards

You will be assessed against the standards expected of a doctor on completion of FY1. Meeting these standards early on in your first year of the Foundation Programme will be difficult, but this is to be expected, as you will of course lack the experience of a doctor at the end of FY1. It is more important that you are able to demonstrate a clear improvement between the beginning and end of the year, enabling you to meet the required standards at the end of FY1.

Collating the results

In June of FY1 or FY2, a collated feedback analysis that brings together the results of all your DOPS, Mini-CEX, CbD and Mini-PAT (if applicable) assessments will be given to you via your educational supervisor. The more assessments you have undertaken that year, the more comprehensive the feedback will be, and the more you should learn about yourself. A comparison sheet for other trainees at your level will also be included.

The thought of all these assessments may be somewhat daunting, but current foundation doctors have responded positively. The immediate feedback gives a sense of achievement, and by giving positive comments, constructive criticism and an agreed plan of action, it helps to shape the Personal Development Plan (PDP).

Box 5.7 provides a list of helpful tips regarding the assessments.

Box 5.7: Assessment tips

- Remember that it is you who has to initiate the assessments. With the exception of MSF, you won't be prompted.
- Opportunities to do assessments, particularly DOPS and Mini-CEX, will occur on a regular basis. Keep your forms handy so that you can take advantage if an opportunity presents itself.
- You don't have to wait for an opportunity to come up – make your own breaks! For example, ask a senior colleague to observe you clerking a new patient on call, or ask a GP if you can see the next patient.
- You can't repeat procedures for multiple DOPS assessments, but no one has said you can't be observed and given feedback a few times in preparation. Ask senior colleagues to observe you and give you informal feedback – they are obliged to help junior doctors.
- Don't worry if you perform badly on an assessment. By the end of the year, you'll be able to show how much you have improved.
- Don't forget that at least one of each type of assessment on each placement should be with the supervising consultant.
- Always check with the patient that it's OK if someone observes you taking their history, examining them and/or performing a procedure.
- Vary your assessors, cases and procedures – repetition will be picked up on.
- Spread your assessments out – don't put undue pressure on yourself or others by leaving them all to the last minute.
- Get *all* of the assessments done and the forms handed in *before* the deadline (around mid-May). Not doing so is a probity issue, as the forms cheerfully remind you.
- Don't fold the forms more than once, as they need to be computer scanned.
- Ensure that the writing goes through all the carbon copies!

Foundation Learning Portfolio

An intimidating-looking item handed to you at induction, your *Foundation Learning Portfolio*[11] will contain all that you need in order to manage your placements and monitor your progress during the Foundation Programme. It will contain guidance and suggestions for gathering evidence, and will be where you keep copies of your assessments, reflective pieces and feedback from others. It goes without saying that it is a most important article and should be the first thing to be saved from a burning building. When you first collect one, it will contain the following:

1   a list of the competences which should be achieved on completion of the Foundation Programme
2   example forms on which to record meetings with your educational supervisor, reflections on your practice, and self-appraisal
3   an educational agreement, setting out the duties of yourself and your supervisors
4   assessment tools
5   a Personal Development Plan (PDP).

During the two years of the Foundation Programme, you must be assessed on all the competences which come under the headings of the seven principles of good medical practice, as described by the GMC. It is up to you to decide how best to demonstrate each competence, either using one of the assessment tools described above or by other means – for example, writing a reflective piece that illustrates your grasp of one or more particular competences. Some specific competences need to be demonstrated by particular methods. For example, a description of how audit can improve personal performance can only be demonstrated by involvement in such a project. Similarly, competence in resuscitation technique must be demonstrated by gaining a certificate of completion of an intermediate life support course. However, the majority of competences may be demonstrated with one or more of the four assessment tools designed for the Foundation Programme.

If your portfolio is kept up to date, it will serve as a record of achievement in the Foundation Programme. It will enable you to identify your own personal strengths and weaknesses, which should aid you not only with your Personal Development Plan for FY2, but also with your career aspirations.

You must submit your portfolio at the end of each year in order to demonstrate that you have attained the required level of competence to progress in your training. It is taken as evidence that you are up to date and fit to practise. This revalidation is a condition of registration with the GMC.

Box 5.8 shows a suggested list of items to retain in your portfolio.

Box 5.8: Items to keep in your portfolio

- Records of appraisals held with your educational supervisor, detailing your progress, requirements and areas for development.
- Your up-to-date PDP, containing objectives for future learning.
- Your assessment outcomes and feedback.
- A record of all the practical procedures you have performed, observed and taught, and when (you may well need this for Royal College examination logbooks later on).
- Copies of all teaching done and presentations given, with feedback if possible.
- Your up-to-date CV and evidence of your qualifications.
- Details of courses you have attended and any certificates awarded.
- Copies of audit projects with which you have been involved.
- Copies of publications.
- Records of any complaints made against you and their outcomes.
- Food for the soul – thank-you cards, details of difficult patients you have successfully diagnosed or treated, and praise from colleagues (remember only to use hospital numbers, not patient names).

You will by now have realised that not just the so-called work–life balance, but also a work–*portfolio* balance is essential in order to survive the Foundation Programme. Incorporating 'collecting evidence' into everyday life can be challenging, but is not impossible. Box 5.9 provides some suggestions on how to manage your portfolio.

Box 5.9: Tips on how to manage your portfolio

- Little and often is the key to keeping your portfolio fresh. It's all too easy to forget to write down practical procedures or to let your CV stagnate, but you won't thank yourself later!
- Keeping a brief diary of cases seen while on call can be a minimally demanding method of accumulating evidence for reflective practice.
- Don't let the portfolio run your life. It is there to prove to outsiders that you are competent and learning at an acceptable rate, as most doctors undertaking the Foundation Programme will be.

Personal Development Plan

Your PDP is an important part of your Foundation Learning Portfolio, in which you will identify and record your specific learning needs and devise a method of achieving these objectives. It will be based on the self-appraisal tool found in your portfolio.

To identify gaps in knowledge, skills or attitudes to include in your self-appraisal and PDP, the *Curriculum*[2] is the best place to start. Discussion with your educational supervisor should enable you to select which elements are most appropriately worked on in each of your placements. However, the *Curriculum*[2] isn't intended as a restrictive document. For example, skills relating to an embedded 'taster' session that you intend to undertake in FY2 (see below) may be legitimately included in your PDP. You will probably also find that feedback from assessments is a good source of PDP goals.

Achievement of the targets that you set yourself may take a variety of forms. Knowledge gaps may be filled by reading around a subject, and practical skills may be brushed up on by requesting supervision and feedback from a senior member of the team while performing an unfamiliar procedure. Whatever method you use, it is important to choose a realistic one – bearing in mind, for example, the demands on others' time when requesting supervision.

You'll be expected to keep your PDP up to date, recording when you have achieved the goals you set out at the start of each placement. You will review your PDP with your educational supervisor at the beginning and end of each placement. Doing this, and evaluating your progress, should provide you with documentation of your improvement in addition to a well-earned sense of satisfaction. In this respect, it is best to keep your goals and their timeframes both realistic and relevant to you and your patients (*see* Worked example 5.2). You can use the PDP as

---

Worked example 5.2: PDP goal

On a Care of the Older Person placement, FY1 doctor James realised that he was having difficulty administering intravenous injections. He spoke to his educational supervisor and agreed on an entry in his PDP about needing to improve this skill. His plan of action was to ask more experienced colleagues if they would be willing to allow him to perform this procedure if their patients required it, to enable him to practise the skill. After making the entry, James performed the procedure many more times than he would have done. A month later, he demonstrated the skill in a DOPS assessment and was seen to be competent. He recorded this outcome in his PDP.

evidence that you have achieved specific competences. To do this you will need your educational or clinical supervisor to sign the PDP form in the portfolio.

In addition to identifying and achieving goals, your PDP should address the tendency towards 'reflective practice' that the modern NHS has evolved. The late Donald Schön, an influential thinker in the field of reflective professional learning, argued that formal theory is often of no use in solving practical problems.[15] Instead, he suggested that reflection *in* action (learning by applying past experiences to current events as they are happening) and reflection *on* action (thinking back to actions taken and how to learn from the experience) are valuable tools for effective learning. Reflection is now said to be the hallmark of the professional, and is one of the core competences of the *Curriculum*.[2]

In this respect it is appropriate to include personal accounts of your experiences and your reflections on them in your PDP. Debriefings with colleagues and regular feedback also provide opportunities for reflection. As already mentioned, these reflections may be used to demonstrate foundation competences, as well as helping you to focus on how your experiences have affected you, your patients and the healthcare team. You may also be stimulated to consider how situations may have been handled differently, and the difference in outcome that this would have caused. This is of course a personal exercise, and care should be taken to protect the confidential nature of your writings.

End of FY1

By the end of FY1, you will be able to put the knowledge, skills and attitudes that you learned as a student into the practice of medicine. You will be able to recognise and successfully manage common situations, as outlined in the GMC document, *The New Doctor*.[16]

To mark the occasion you will acquire a well-earned 'Certificate of Experience' confirming that you have performed satisfactorily during FY1, and that you have undertaken 3 months of medicine and 3 months of surgery. This is now completed during the application for full registration with the GMC at the end of FY1 (*see* Box 5.10). You will first have to have the Attainment of FY1 Competency form in your portfolio signed off.

Box 5.10: Full GMC registration[1]

1 Download an application form from www.gmc-uk.org and complete the first page with your personal details, leaving the Certificate of Experience on the back page blank.

2 Send the Certificate of Experience, along with the Certificates of Satisfactory Service which you will have received after each post, to your medical school for signature. They will then return the Certificate of Experience to you (or in some cases will send it to the GMC for you – check with your medical school). Note that the person who is to sign the Certificate of Experience must have been sent every Certificate of Satisfactory Service you receive after each FY1 post you undertake. It is your responsibility to ensure that these are received as each post is completed. *Don't* wait until you have finished all 12 months.

3 On receipt of the completed Certificate of Experience, forward it, along with the registration fee (currently £290), to the GMC address on the form, for approval.

4 The GMC normally responds within five working days to acknowledge receipt of the application. Once it has been approved, you will be sent a certificate confirming your full registration, valid from the date when your postgraduate experience was completed.

Note: It is best to send your application as early as possible, well in advance of the date when you will require full registration. At peak times of the year the GMC is overwhelmed by applications, and delays are possible.

Summary

1 The Foundation Programme is the new bridge between medical school and specialist training. It aims to produce doctors who are competent to begin specialist training in any field of medicine.

2 It is a two-year programme that all new doctors in the UK will undertake after graduating from medical school, and it replaces the former PRHO and SHO1 years.

3 Before you start work, make sure that you have been provisionally registered with the GMC, have joined a defence body and are in possession of a job offer, contract and job description.

4 When you start work, you will need to balance your duties as a doctor with training requirements, being a savvy NHS employee and having a life outside medicine. This can be tough, but everyone is in the same boat, so don't be afraid to ask for help.

5 FY1 consists of a variety of placements, so use them to start planning your career from the word go. Use the portfolio and PDP, but remember that you are your own best resource.

6 At the end of FY1, you will receive a Certificate of Experience, and will be eligible for full registration with the GMC.

References

1   General Medical Council website; www.gmc-uk.org
2   *Curriculum for the Foundation Years in Postgraduate Education and Training*; www.mmc.nhs.uk
3   *Operational Framework for Foundation Training*; www.mmc.nhs.uk
4   Donaldson L. *Unfinished Business*. London: Department of Health; 2002.
5   Sanders S, Dawson J, Datta S *et al. The Oxford Handbook for the Foundation Programme*. New York: Oxford University Press; 2005.
6   Urmston I. Are you about to start as a preregistration house officer? *studentBMJ.* 2001; **9:** 1946; www.studentbmj.com/back_issues/0601/careers/194.html
7   *The Junior Doctors' Handbook*, produced annually by the BMA and available to view in the members-only sections of the BMA website (www.bma.org.uk) and the *studentBMJ* website (www.studentbmj.com).
8   British Medical Association website; www.bma.org.uk
9   Urmston I. Starting house jobs on the right footing. *studentBMJ.* 2002; **10:** 215–58; www.studentbmj.com/issues/02/07/editorials/216.php
10 *Rough Guide to the Foundation Programme*; www.mmc.nhs.uk
11 *Foundation Learning Portfolio*; www.mmc.nhs.uk
12 *Pay Scales for Doctors 2006*; www.nhscareers.nhs.uk/nhs-knowledge_base/data/5340.html
13 *Good Medical Practice*; www.gmc-uk.org/guidance/good_medical_practice/index.asp
14 Foundation Assessment section on Healthcare Assessment & Training website; www.hcat.nhs.uk/foundation
15 Schön DA. *Educating the Reflective Practitioner: toward a new design for teaching and learning in the professions.* San Francisco, CA: Jossey-Bass; 1987.
16 The New Doctor; www.gmc-uk.org/education/foundation/new_doctor.asp

Further reading

• Pilot results for the Foundation Programme; www.mmc.nhs.uk

Chapter 6

FY2 and beyond

Introduction to FY2

Whereas the GMC is responsible for the education of FY1 doctors, in FY2 the responsibility falls to the recently formed Postgraduate Medical Education and Training Board (PMETB). This body will not only set the standards of training for FY2, but will also oversee specialty and GP training and beyond.

The second year of foundation training aims to build on FY1, and to equip foundation doctors with the generic skills that they will require in order to successfully practise medicine regardless of specialty. Such generic competences include teamworking, communication and consultation skills, effective time management, patient safety, IT skills and the use of evidence and data. FY2 will also focus on the assessment and management of the acutely ill patient, to ensure that all doctors will be safe in an emergency.

Structure of FY2

The second foundation year will normally consist of three 4-month placements in a variety of specialties, as described in the *Rough Guide*.[1] In addition, it may be possible for your educational supervisor to arrange with you one or more 'taster' sessions, in which you would work for a different specialty for a week to give you a feel for other particular areas of expertise. This provides an excellent opportunity to gain first-hand experience of a broad range of specialties, which is one of the main aims of the Foundation Programme.

The specific placements that you will undertake in FY2 may or may not be known to you at the start of your foundation training, and the method of FY2 allocation at your particular foundation school will have a bearing on the placements that you are able to undertake. Different schools will employ different means of allocating foundation doctors to FY2 placements. Some will take into account preferences for FY2 at the admission stage of the Foundation Programme, allowing trainees to know from the outset the content and location of their placements in both years. However, other schools will encourage trainees to express their preferences approximately 6 to 8 months into FY1, following discussion with educational supervisors.

Whichever method is used, the element of choice should not be overstated. Due to the finite nature of posts available for foundation doctors, there will always be oversubscribed specialties, which means that not every applicant will get their first choice. Rest assured, however, that the combinations of placements are carefully devised by each school in order to maximise the range of experiences that each trainee will have, thus ensuring that all doctors will be able to achieve the required FY2 competences. One would assume that it is not the foundation schools' intention to hinder a number of medical graduates after so many thousands of pounds of taxpayers' money have been spent on their basic medical education!

The other concern is that FY2 placements might have a bearing on the chances of getting into a particular specialty after foundation training, but this suggestion has been refuted by MMC. Given that FY2 allocations are not made strictly on the basis of merit, it would certainly be unjust to use them as a prerequisite for entry to particular specialist training. However, the placements that you undertake might well interest you career-wise in a specialty you had not considered before – so, free from the pressure of competing for placements that incorporate your perceived 'chosen' specialty, you can open your eyes to a range of other fields.

The curriculum in FY2

While the FY2 year builds on the competences acquired during FY1 in accordance with 'spiral' learning, it also focuses on the identification and care of the acutely unwell patient. And as the management of chronic disease is an ever-growing area of medicine, the relationship between this and the presentation of acute illness will also be a theme of FY2. At least one of your FY2 posts should allow experience in an acute care setting.

By the end of FY2 you will be ready to start specialist training, and you will be professionally accountable for patient safety. To this end, FY2 will also concentrate on taking responsibility for the care of your patients.

Formal teaching in FY2

As in FY1, there is a structured teaching programme in FY2, this time taking place over 10 days of study leave. This generic professional training will include the development of transferable skills such as teamwork, communication skills and decision making, as well as managing complaints, using evidence, ethics and law, and teaching and appraisal. Most FY2 doctors will also be expected to undertake a supervised clinical audit project during this time. This is a project examining a current practice in order to compare that practice with a set standard, such as a guideline. If current practice differs from the desired standard, the cause is pinpointed and suggestions for rectifying it are made before the audit is repeated.

You will also be eligible for up to another 20 days' study leave, which should be used to attend courses away from the clinical setting or to find out about careers that you haven't had the opportunity to sample thus far. This might be done in the form of embedded 'taster' days or mini-placements in areas of interest to you (see the section on FY2 placements below). FY2 study leave is not intended for studying for specialist examinations, as these are now aimed at doctors after the first two postgraduate years (i.e. in the second year of SHO level or beyond). These exams don't count in the context of entry to the first two years of specialist training, and so taking on the extra work at this stage isn't recommended! Royal College membership will almost certainly be a requirement later on, in the third year of specialist training. More information is available on the MMC website.

Many postgraduate courses are available to occupy your study leave, and the details of several are listed on the BMA website. It is usually best to try to find someone who has already undertaken a particular course, or a senior colleague who recommends it, rather than taking a gamble – especially as many of these courses involve considerable expense. You may be entitled to claim expenses for travel and subsistence relating to courses taken during study leave, but you must meet the cost of any examinations taken yourself.

Study leave should be planned as far in advance as possible – you may have to swap on-calls, which is easiest done early.

FY2 placements

The new placements available to trainees in FY2 fall into three categories – shortage specialties, general practice and academic medicine. You will need to find out what placements are available at your particular foundation school. Entry into FY2 placements will be particularly competitive in the case of stand-alone, non-2-year programmes.

Shortage specialties

Several medical specialties are actively recruiting, and to this end additional funding has been made available to offer FY2 placements in these areas in order to spark the interest of young doctors. Although the availability of placements will vary, there is likely to be a broad selection in most programmes.

This may seem like a thinly veiled way in which to shunt junior doctors into the less popular specialties, but it is also intended to help you to make career decisions. You may come across a specialty that interests you and decide to go for it, rather than enduring vicious competition for the field in which you always thought you wanted to specialise.

Box 6.1 lists some of the current shortage specialties.

Box 6.1: Shortage specialties

These specialties, and others, are likely to be on offer for FY2 placements:

- allergy
- audiological medicine
- chemical pathology/metabolic medicine
- clinical genetics
- critical care/intensive-care medicine
- genito-urinary medicine
- histopathology
- immunology
- medical microbiology
- nuclear medicine
- psychiatry
- public health medicine
- radiology
- virology.

General practice

A stint of practising medicine in the community after several months of secondary care experience will provide a refreshing change for many. While learning to care for patients in their own environment, you will see illness in much earlier stages of development and will be prompted to consider more deeply the socio-economic factors that come into play in the lives of your patients. The management of these patients will take on a different form, incorporating a measure of risk assessment, as well as consideration of the patient's role in the community. The experience should allow you to develop a greater appreciation of your patients as people, not just walking illnesses that require treatment. You will also gain a better insight into the relationship between primary and secondary care. This appreciation is what you should work towards as a foundation trainee in general practice – the placement will not be designed to train you as a general practitioner.

In terms of working patterns, general practice will provide you with experience of operating within a relatively small team, and there will potentially be opportunities for one-to-one learning on a regular basis. A trained supervisor will be working with you to help you to maximise the learning potential of the placement. On average, an FY2 doctor will spend six half-days each week seeing patients while working with GPs and other members of the extended primary healthcare team. The remainder of the time will be allocated to structured teaching at the foundation school, completing assessments, project work and work-based teaching, making for a full but varied timetable.

General practice placements have proved to be a popular part of pilot programmes, with a significant proportion of trainees expressing an interest in entering this field as a career. Seeing patients alone and taking part in home visits have been cited by trainees in London[2] as having a positive effect on their personal confidence. Foundation doctors also come away with a better appreciation of effective correspondence between doctors in primary and secondary care, and a less lax approach to the ordering of investigations.

MMC claimed that just over half of the first cohort of doctors entering FY2 (in August 2006) were expected to undertake a placement in general practice, with the figure apparently staying the same or even rising the following year. This is designed to support the NHS drive to increasingly shift the 'patient experience' into primary care, lessening the work and financial burden of secondary care on the service.

Academic medicine

'Academic medicine' is an umbrella term for the use of a medical degree to delve into research or education. Academics lead a research team and teach in addition to their clinical responsibilities. Placements in this area during the Foundation Programme will be useful for those considering this career path.

There are currently two ways of incorporating academic medicine into the early postgraduate years of a medical career. For those candidates who are relatively confident about their career aspirations, a fully integrated clinical and research attachment based in a single department is available, which can last either one or two years. This placement allows doctors to continue to see patients and work towards common foundation competences while at the same time honing their research skills. On completion of the Foundation Programme the candidate may then apply for a clinical fellowship. This type of programme may suit MBBS PhD graduates, who have already expressed a strong interest in research.

Alternatively, it is possible to apply for 4-month placements in academic departments, as one of the FY2 posts. This option is more suitable for exploring potential interests in the field.

Whatever foundation placements you undertake, it is likely that your department will be involved in research in one way or another. It is always worth talking to the consultant and exploring opportunities to get involved. If you don't ask, you don't get!

After the Foundation Programme, promising academics may choose to pursue a full- or part-time taught (e.g. MSc) or research (e.g. PhD) degree. Recently it was announced that doctors working towards such a higher degree whilst at SHO level may apply to defer their entry into specialist training for up to three years in order to complete their research; further guidance can be found on the MMC website. More information on academic medicine, including a downloadable copy of *A Pocket Guide to Academic Training Opportunities,* can also be found on the MMC website.[3]

'Taster' experiences

In your study leave during FY2 you may wish to 'have a go' at a specialty that is not included in your foundation placements for a week or two. This is a way of informing your career aspirations and exploring your potential, as well as getting an idea of the specialty's contribution to patient care. There may be such placements complete with trainee timetables – already set up in some trusts, but in most cases the starting point is to discuss the idea with your educational supervisor.

A draft template for embedded tasters can be found in Appendix 7 of the *Framework.*[4] Personal accounts of specific tasters in various fields are available on the MMC website.

Assessments and portfolios in FY2

The official introduction of the assessment tools into FY2 took place in August 2006, as the first intake of foundation doctors moved into the second year of the programme. At the time of writing, the signs indicate that the same assessment methods that are used in FY1 will also be employed in FY2, but a greater number of assessments will need to be undertaken. They will be assessed at the standard that a doctor should have achieved at the end of the Foundation Programme.

The assessments are again an important method of monitoring your progress and providing you with feedback as the year goes on. Your postgraduate dean will use the assessment results to judge your satisfactory completion of the programme and grant the award of a Foundation Achievement of Competency Document (FACD), which indicates that you have completed the programme.

In addition to your assessments, your portfolio will also contain your PDP for FY2, educational agreements, reflective pieces and records of meetings with your educational supervisor.

The end of FY2

As you draw towards the end of your second year in the Foundation Programme, you will be taking on increasing levels of responsibility and accountability for patient care.

Once you have finished all of your foundation assessments to a good standard, the FACD in your portfolio will be signed off to show that your foundation training is complete. You will now be able to follow your chosen career path.

Specialist and GP training programmes

Changes to the system

The previous system of specialist training was fraught with problems. A bottleneck between SHO and SpR levels was maintained by the former waiting around for higher posts, as there was no defined end-point to training. Coupled with poor availability of careers advice and no formal system of assessment or appraisal, a high percentage of doctors languished in junior positions for years before moving up the career ladder. This was a major factor prompting a high percentage of doctors to leave medicine two years or more after graduation.

There has been much debate over the reorganisation of training after the Foundation Programme, and the four UK Health Departments only recently agreed (in the summer of 2006) on a new career framework for life after the Foundation Programme.

Post-foundation training is being redeveloped by the PMETB and the Royal Colleges with the aim of combining the basic specialist training of the traditional SHO post and the SpR-level advanced training. This should extend the system of structured curricula and assessment previously only employed at SpR level to all stages of training. The programmes will initially be broadly based, and will become more focused as time goes on. They will take doctors right through to consultant level, at which point they will achieve a Certificate of Completion of Training (CCT). To this end, the training is also known as 'run-through' training.

In fact, so drastic is the overhaul that name changes (albeit small ones) have been commissioned. The titles of SpR and SHO will be no more from January and August 2007 respectively (apart from those already in the jobs). The end of January 2007 will see the start of recruitment to Specialty Registrar (StR) training programmes, more on which can be found on the MMC website.

MMC has many good intentions concerning the redevelopment of specialty training. As with the Foundation Programme, it is hoped that training will be streamlined and doctors will be 'judgment safe' in their ability to identify and care for acutely ill patients. Communication skills and patient choice are other foci of the training. MMC also wants to see opportunities within specialties for 'supra-specialisation', which it hopes will have a large enough degree of flexibility to allow training to accommodate advances in medical technology and alterations in service demands. Happily for doctors, it is hoped that there will be improved opportunities for career breaks, and fairness and equality in the workplace will be monitored.

New curricula are being devised for each specialty, and these will provide a framework of standards against which doctors will be assessed. The length of specialty training programmes will be determined on an individual basis by the PMETB, the medical Royal Colleges and the specialties themselves, to reflect the individual curricula for each specialty. For example, general practice will require three years' specialist training, whereas other fields may require up to seven years.

Applying for specialist training

About halfway through FY2, you will need to make decisions about which career path to follow. However, this does not mean that you should wait until then to start thinking about your career! Entry to specialties (either general practice or secondary care specialties) will be by open and fair competition, and you are likely to stand a better chance of success if you have made an informed application on the basis of not only your interests, but also your aptitudes and a realistic assessment of employment opportunities. 'Taster' experiences should help to inform your preferences, but be aware that a long and arduous road often lies ahead for those with just one career in mind.

Other points to bear in mind when applying are that the placements you undertook during the Foundation Programme have no bearing on selection for run-through training, and that there are currently no plans to use foundation training performance in the selection process. However, assessment results may be considered for use in future years. Trainees will be notified at the beginning of their programme if this is to be the case for their cohort.

A timeline for recruitment into specialty training has been made available on the MMC website, and confirms that the process will be a national one, again administered by MTAS. Doctors will be able to apply to either one or two 'specialty groups' (about 16 groups which contain all the specialties; further details are due to be published on the MMC and MTAS websites), and can choose one or two locations (apart from in General Practice). Details of programmes and job descriptions will be available on the deanery websites in December, ready for the short window for receipt of applications around the end of January.

Shortlisting and interviews will be conducted locally using a nationally-agreed set of criteria for each specialty. You will, of course, be pitted against doctors of similar competence and experience for entry. This means that as the new system is being phased in, current SHOs will be able to apply to later years in run-through training programmes, while Foundation Programme leavers will enter the first year. Two rounds of recruitment will take place, with the results of both being announced through the MTAS website.

If your application for a specialist training programme is unsuccessful, you will be able to apply for a fixed-term specialist training appointment (FTSTA) lasting one year. As mentioned in Chapter 1, these are posts which train Foundation Programme leavers to the same standard as the first year of the run-through training programme, but which leave doctors at a loose end at the end of the year. At this point, you may reapply for run-through training in the specialty or apply for another FTSTA.

How it will work

Run-through training posts are currently advertised towards the end of the year, with doctors competing for entry during a process of short-listing and selection between the months of February and June. The general timescale of the application process is expected to remain similar in later years.

Once they have been accepted on to a run-through training pro-gramme, doctors will start that programme directly after FY2, taking on the new title of StR as they do so. The goal to work towards now will be a Certificate of Completion of Training (CCT), and the time taken to reach this level will vary between specialties.

On attainment of a CCT, you will be eligible to be entered on the Specialist or GP Register, and can then apply for a senior medical appointment (GP, consultant, or other specialist role). Doctors who have not completed a training programme to achieve a CCT may apply to the PMETB for entry to the Specialist Register (for example, doctors who have considerable experience but who are in non-training career posts rather than specialty training appointments).

During run-through training, doctors will usually attempt the exam-inations for Royal College membership. The first step is to contact the appropriate Royal College and ask for a copy of the examination pre-requisites (*see* Chapter 8). Most College examinations consist of two parts, roughly speaking – basic science and clinical skills. Preparation for each part normally takes six months, and a gap of a year between taking the parts is the norm.[5]

Summary

1   FY2 will give you the opportunity to broaden your horizons by working in a variety of specialties. Time in shortage specialties and general practice is encouraged, and there are opportunities to break into academic medicine.
2   All FY2 leavers should be confident in their ability to care appropriately for acutely ill patients and to take responsibility for the care of these patients.
3   Not doing a foundation placement in a specialty that interests you will not prohibit you from applying for specialist training in that field. 'Taster' experiences can be arranged for you to test your affinity for other fields.
4   At the end of FY2, you will receive a FACD and will be ready to begin specialist training. This will involve you working towards a CCT, which will eventually enable you to join the Specialist or GP Register and apply for a senior appointment.

References

1   *Rough Guide to the Foundation Programme;* www.mmc.nhs.uk
2   Firth-Cozens J. *The Patient Journey: the London Pilot of the primary care experience;* www.mmc.nhs.uk
3   Information pertaining to academic medicine can be found at www.mmc.nhs.uk
4   *Operational Framework for Foundation Training;* www.mmc.nhs.uk
5   Sanders S, Dawson J, Datta S *et al. The Oxford Handbook for the Foundation Programme.* New York: Oxford University Press; 2005.

Further reading

- MMC policy documents; www.mmc.nhs.uk
- *MMC Career Framework Explained;* www.mmc.nhs.uk

Chapter 7

Frequently asked questions

Applying to the Foundation Programme

Am I guaranteed a job in my home foundation school?

You wish! There are enough jobs for all UK graduates, but not necessarily in the location of their choice. However, it's worth pointing out that 70% of students got a job in one of their top ten choices in MDAP, so if you keep away from the competitive areas, the chances are that you'll be OK.

Are the achievements that we list on our application form checked?

Applications will be randomly selected for checks, so don't even think about fabricating achievements. Lying is a big no-no for doctors, and making something up on this form could see you hauled up in front of the GMC for a fitness-to-practise hearing. Every single achievement that you list on your form should be something you can back up with material evidence – so if you talk about playing for the rugby team, a team photo will be ample evidence. It's also worth bearing in mind that the trust which offers you a job can ask for evidence, so the need for proof doesn't end after MTAS!

You're saying not to apply to London, but I want to become a big professor, so surely I need to be working in the capital's prestigious hospitals as early as I can?

All right, calm down! The fact is, half of those people starting specialist training in London have never previously worked in the capital, so you've got plenty of time to apply after the foundation years. You'll stand a better chance of getting a London job at this stage, too.

The opportunity to do an intercalated degree is limited only to the very highest achievers at my medical school. Not being able to do one means I'm screwed, doesn't it?

Not at all. Intercalated degrees are optional, so there are no marks set aside for them.

I'm a graduate with a mortgage and a family. Surely I'll get the job of my choice?

Not necessarily. But the aim of this isn't to break up families, so these things will definitely be taken into account – but there are no guarantees.

But what about me and my girlfriend? We're in the final year together and we don't want to be apart!

Ah! Unfortunately, MTAS is a loveless demon who recognises not this human emotion you call 'love'. Your best bet is to apply to the same places together and, if working in the same region is of the utmost importance to you, consider applying to less competitive UoAs where the chances are you'll both get in.

Financial constraints mean that I was only able to arrange an elective within the UK. This is going to make me look less attractive on the MTAS form when compared with others, isn't it?

Nope – an elective isn't a competition to see who can get the most tropical diseases. You'll learn plenty if you do an elective in the UK, and those marking the form don't make any distinction according to elective location, so don't be afraid to write about it!

It's ridiculous expecting us to talk about non-academic achievements when we're applying for medical jobs!

Well, you have to mention them on applications for any other job in any other career. Get out of your bubble, man!

What happens if after I've been allocated to a UoA I'm allocated a job I don't like?

Grin and bear it, I'm afraid. You can get into serious trouble if you turn down a job, so it's certainly not something we recommend.

The academic Foundation Programme looks pretty hot to me, but in all honesty I'm not sure I want to become an academic at the end of it. Is that OK?

Of course it is, Professor! You won't be forced to move into the game if you don't want to. The point of the programme is to give people a chance to try academia out and see if it's the sort of thing they like.

Damn it, I missed out on a place on the academic Foundation Programme. My childhood dreams of being a professor of anal medicine are gone now, right?

Worry not, young padawan, you'll have plenty of other opportunities to enter academic medicine. Academia is a field into which the medical profession needs to recruit more people, so MMC aims to make it easier for you to get into it, not harder!

Why don't the jobs list information on banding, consultants and holidays?

This information changes too frequently for it to be included. It's annoying, but if people made decisions on the basis of this information and then it changed, they'd be even more annoyed!

The Foundation Programme

Can I defer the start of the Foundation Programme?

This is possible under certain circumstances, but these must be convincing. Undertaking a BSc might constitute a good reason, but a year of celebrating the end of medical school would not!

In the case of a two-year Foundation Programme, permission must be sought from the postgraduate dean or director of the foundation school by which you have been accepted, at least three months before the start of the Foundation Programme. You cannot normally defer the programme for more than one year. Stand-alone FY1 or FY2 posts that are not part of a two-year programme can only be deferred in exceptional situations.

Is it possible for overseas doctors to enter FY2 without completing FY1?

In April 2006, regulations came into force whereby all international medical graduates (IMGs) will be excluded from appointment to training posts after FY2, unless the recruiting trust can prove that there are no suitably qualified UK or European Economic Area (EEA) applicants for the post in question. This shock ruling, announced by the Department of Health without consultation with doctors' organisations such as the BMA, the medical Royal Colleges or overseas doctors' associations, is unfortunately likely to discourage many IMGs from seeking a career in the UK. At the time of writing, several students' and doctors' groups are campaigning for fair debate of the legislation and provisions for those already working in the country.

However, it is still possible for overseas doctors to apply for entry to the UK's Foundation Programme, with entry to either year being theoretically possible. It is not necessary for doctors who are eligible for limited or full GMC registration to complete FY1 before entry to FY2. However, since most FY2 posts will be taken up by FY1 doctors moving up in the system, competition for any spare posts is likely to be fierce. These posts will be advertised in the national medical press (such as *BMJ Careers*), and possibly locally by individual deaneries or trusts, in the first few months of the year. Deaneries and foundation schools are actively looking to create additional FY2 posts that would provide a suitable entry point for overseas doctors.

It is advisable for overseas doctors to glean all of the available information and advice from the NHS, GMC and Department of Health before applying for a post in the UK.

Am I entitled to maternity leave within the Foundation Programme?

All new mothers are entitled to 26 weeks' paid maternity leave, after which they must be permitted to return to work. If you have been in employment for 6 months or more, you can apply for another 26 weeks' unpaid leave. New fathers who have worked for over 6 months are entitled to 2 weeks' paid leave. Whether the employment has to have been with one particular trust or just with the NHS is unclear. More information can be found in the *Junior Doctors' Handbook*.

Can I train part-time in the Foundation Programme?

It is possible to train part-time as a foundation doctor on at least a half-time basis if you have a valid reason for doing so. The main reasons are disability or ill health and caring for a child, an ill or disabled partner, a relative or some other dependant. A full list of valid reasons will be available from your deanery.

You do not need to state your intention to train part-time on your application form, but you should discuss it with your postgraduate deanery in order to confirm your eligibility. You should inform the foundation school that accepts you as soon as possible so that they can make arrangements. This will usually mean either sharing an educational post (*not* a job) with another trainee, or reducing the number of hours in a full-time post.

Training part-time does of course mean that your foundation training will be extended, as you must still complete the equivalent of two years' full-time training before you can achieve a FACD. This remains the case even if you meet the required competences early.

Can I take time out of the Foundation Programme?

Again the answer is yes, but you need a good reason. Health, personal and domestic reasons may be acceptable, as well as working or travelling abroad. You will need to discuss the possibility of time out with your educational supervisor in the first instance.

Once you have made the decision, you will need to complete a 'Time Out of Foundation Programme' form, which is available from your

Foundation Programme Training Director (FPTD) and should be returned to them by the end of the sixth month of FY1. In the absence of exceptional circumstances you will usually only be permitted to take a one-year break (i.e. the year that would have been your FY2).

Six months before your return, you will need to complete an FY2 placement preference form so that a placement will be available for you at the start of the academic year. If you fail to do this, you will have to apply competitively for an FY2 post.

Is there any way that I can change deaneries once I've started the Foundation Programme?

This is difficult, but not impossible. You will need a good reason, such as carer responsibilities, health concerns or the pursuit of research opportunities, and you will normally only be able to transfer at the start of FY1 or FY2. In addition, the request has to be agreed upon by your FPTD, postgraduate dean and the new deanery, and there must obviously be a place available at the new deanery.

If you are not eligible for an inter-deanery transfer, you can take a gamble and give notice to your current trust and withdraw from your current deanery in order to apply to a different one for an advertised FY2 post. This is a risky approach, and you should discuss it with your FPTD and educational supervisor, as well as your postgraduate dean.

Can I train abroad as part of the Foundation Programme?

It is possible for training outside the UK to count towards your acquisition of foundation competences in FY2, provided that certain conditions are met. The PMETB currently requires that the training abroad will address the specific foundation competences, will use competency-based assessment methods, and has been agreed upon by the postgraduate dean who has recommended it to the PMETB for approval.

The *Operational Framework* has more information on training abroad within the foundation years.

In addition, the BMA publishes *Working Abroad: a guide for BMA members* and *Opportunities for Doctors in the EEA*, both available on the website at www.bma.org.uk. These resources provide country-specific advice, legislation and other useful information. Seminars on working abroad are held by the BMA (for further information, contact the BMA's International Department on 020 7383 6491).

I'm being bullied/harassed at work. What can I do?

The trust that you work for will have a policy on these issues, and the Human Resources department will be able to advise you on this. Your deanery or foundation school will also have a policy. Both bodies have a responsibility to ensure that bullying and harassment are not tolerated under any circumstances. If you are a BMA member, you can also use their 24-hour telephone counselling service in confidence, on 08459 200169. A career in medicine is stressful enough without putting up with this.

I already know which field I wish to specialise in. Can I work in this field in both FY1 and FY2?

Foundation Programmes with the content of both years known at the outset should not contain experience in the same field twice, and it is not recommended that you choose similar FY1 and FY2 placements if you are completing the years separately. The reason for this is that one of the fundamental aims of the Foundation Programme is to give trainees as broad an experience of medicine as possible. You would be doing yourself a disservice by limiting your options at such an early stage, when breadth of experience and attainment of basic competences are paramount. Every specialty that you spend time in adds another string to your bow, as it were, ensuring that you can demonstrate all of the required skills, attitudes and knowledge by the end of FY2. And of course your career plans may change and leave you at a disadvantage later on. It is best to keep your options open.

I've been allocated a GP placement in a tiny practice. How will I complete the assessments with such a small pool of potential assessors?

In general practice placements or small hospitals this situation may occasionally arise. 'Recycling' of assessors will undoubtedly be flagged up on submission of your assessment forms, but if you can demonstrate that this was only out of necessity you should be given some leeway. In the Mini-PAT, scientific and administrative colleagues (the latter only in general practice) may be nominated as assessors, but should not answer any questions pertaining to your clinical performance. Unfortunately, no matter how desperate you are, you can't be assessed using the DOPS, Mini-CEX or CbD tools by other foundation doctors!

Where can I find more information about the assessments?

Sample assessment forms, guidance, training videos and tables of specific competences to which the assessment tools pertain can be found on the *Health Care Assessment and Training* (*HCAT*) website (www.hcat.nhs.uk/foundation). Descriptions of the standards that you should be attaining in each competency can be found on the same site under the heading 'Assessor written training' in the section for each tool.

What should I do if I have a problem with the assessments?

If you have a query or problem, your educational supervisor should be your first port of call. Information is also available at www.mmc.nhs.uk. In addition, you can speak to your administrator or FPTD. Don't panic if you are struggling with the assessments – there are measures in place to help you, provided that you seek help early enough. Additional assessments, focused training and extensions to the programme will be made available to those who require them. Details can be found in the *Curriculum*.

What happens if I fail one of the foundation years?

The vast majority of trainees are expected to pass these years, and support will be available for those who recognise that they are struggling before it comes to failing one of the years, so don't worry too much.

However, if you do fail FY1, you will not be eligible for full registration with the GMC and you will not be able to enter FY2. In this case you will be given support and allowed up to an extra 12 months to attain the competences for FY1. If you still don't come up to scratch, you will be expected to stop practising medicine.

A similar arrangement will exist for FY2, whereby failing trainees will be given an extension to their training for a stated period of time, normally 6 months. In exceptional circumstances, a further 6 months may be granted. If you do not fulfil the requirements within this extra time, you will not receive a FACD and you may have to stop practising medicine.

Rather than worrying unduly about failure, it is best to recognise when problems are developing and to seek help early enough. Your assessment results will help you to identify problems, and your educational adviser should be available to help you to rectify them.

If I pass all the assessments before time, can I finish the Foundation Programme early?

If you satisfy the clinical competences prior to the end of FY2, you may be able to undertake a short research project or clinical audit in the remaining time. Your educational supervisor will be able to advise you on this. All placements in both FY1 and FY2 must be completed in order to acquire the FACD, so it is not possible to finish the Foundation Programme early.

Chapter 8

Useful resources

Careers advice

- www.mtas.nhs.uk – not strictly a careers advice resource but get familiar with this baby as it's the website you'll need to log on to to apply to foundation year jobs.
- Deanery/foundation school careers advisers – an obvious start!
- Clinical and educational supervisors may be able to give you advice pertaining to their particular specialty.
- The BMA and BMJ Careers (www.bmjcareers.com), BMJ Careers Advice Zone (www.bmjcareersadvicezone.synergynewmedia.co.uk) – job advertisements, career tips, FAQs, links. More information than you can shake a stethoscope at.
- NHS Careers (www.nhscareers.nhs.uk) – juicy careers in the NHS, mmm … tasty.
- Postgraduate deanery websites (www.mmc.nhs.uk) – available specialty training places. Useful, but also good reading for insomniacs.
- MMC (www.mmc.nhs.uk) – the exciting, exhilarating, fascinating latest developments in postgraduate education.
- PMETB (www.pmetb.org.uk) – postgraduate medical education-type stuff. Useful information but bad photographs of happy young doctors.
- BMA (www.bma.org.uk) – 'Careers guidance' section of website. More useful information and all-round more pleasing photographs of happy young doctors. You will feel happier just looking at them. The BMA also holds careers fairs and publishes *Medical Specialties: the way forward*, for a spot of bedtime reading.
- Royal Society of Medicine (www.rsm.ac.uk) – wow, another website with more advice – what are the chances? But this one's royal, so wear a hat.
- Support for Doctors (www.support4doctors.org/default.asp) – set up by the Royal Benevolent Medical Fund. More of that good nourishing advice on careers, money and welfare.
- Doctors.net (www.doctors.net.uk) – spiffing news and education site with an active forum, only accessible to those registered at a UK medical school or with a GMC number.
- London Deanery's Career Guide (www.londondeanery.ac.uk/Career-Guide) – careers information from the London Deanery, offering detailed information on over 50 specialties … and free bagels, maybe.
- *Medical Student Newspaper* (www.medical-student.co.uk) – monthly newspaper for London's medical students, but with general information, too. The world's greatest medical student publication. Probably – no, definitely.
- Taster experiences – not the free wine and cheese ones, but areas of medicine and surgery that interest you. They're designed for you to test-run different areas, so take advantage of them.

- Your portfolio – think about your strengths and weaknesses, and bear in mind the competition. You're the best – never forget that. The force will be with you, always.

Useful organisations

Defence organisations

These provide medico-legal advice, support and representation to medical professionals. You must be a member of one by the time you start your first job. Freebies are usually on offer to medical student members, whose membership is also free.

Medical Defence Union (MDU)
Tel: 020 7202 1500
Website: www.the-mdu.com
Email: mdu@the-mdu.com

Medical Protection Society (MPS)
Tel: 0845 605 4000
Website: www.medicalprotection.org/Medical/United_Kingdom
Email: info@mps.org.uk

Medical and Dental Defence Union of Scotland (MDDUS)
Tel: 0141 221 5858
Website: www.mddus.com
Email: info@mddus.com

British Medical Association (BMA)

The UK doctors' trade union, and sole organisation with negotiating rights for doctors. The BMA campaigns on doctors' behalf, sends its members the weekly *British Medical Journal (BMJ)*, and provides advice in cases of difficulties with employers.

Tel: 0870 606 0828 (*ask*BMA, the information and advice service for members of the organisation)
Website: www.bma.org.uk
Email: via feedback form from the website

General Medical Council (GMC)

The GMC oversees medical education up to the end of FY1, and is responsible for providing the public with competent doctors. To maintain high standards among doctors working in the UK, all must gain registration with the GMC, and therefore all must complete the Foundation Programme, which has been based on the GMC's requirements.

Tel: 0845 357 3456
Website: www.gmc-uk.org
Email: gmc@gmc-uk.org

Postgraduate Medical Education and Training Board (PMETB)

Established in 2005, PMETB does exactly what it says on the tin. It is responsible for setting the UK's standards for postgraduate medical education, starting with FY2. It ensures that all doctors listed on the Specialist Register and the Register of General Practitioners have attained the required level of competence. It is also charged, along with the medical Royal Colleges, with the design of new specialist training programmes.

Tel: 0871 220 3070
Website: www.pmetb.org.uk
Email: info@pmetb.org.uk

Income protection

Companies such as Medical Sickness provide customers with income protection in case of illness.

Tel: 0800 358 6060
Website: www.medical-sickness.co.uk
Email: via form on website

Royal Colleges

The websites of the Royal Colleges provide an insight into what the different specialties involve, along with their requirements and advice.

Royal College of Physicians; www.rcplondon.ac.uk
Royal College of Physicians and Surgeons of Glasgow; www.rcpsglasg. ac.uk

Royal College of Surgeons of England; www.rcseng.ac.uk
Royal College of Surgeons of Edinburgh; www.rcsed.ac.uk
Royal College of Anaesthetists; www.rcoa.ac.uk
Royal College of General Practitioners; www.rcgp.org.uk
Royal College of Obstetricians and Gynaecologists; www.rcog.org.uk
Royal College of Ophthalmologists; www.rcophth.ac.uk
Royal College of Paediatrics and Child Health; www.rcpch.ac.uk
Royal College of Pathologists; www.rcpath.org
Royal College of Psychiatrists; www.rcpsych.ac.uk
Royal College of Radiologists; www.rcr.ac.uk

UK deaneries and foundation schools

1   Northern Ireland; www.nimdta.gov.uk
2   Scotland; www.mmc.scot.nhs.uk
3   Wales; www.cardiff.ac.uk/pgmde
4   Northern Deanery; http://mypimd.ncl.ac.uk/PIMD_new2
5   Yorkshire Deanery; www.yorkshiredeanery.com
6   North Western Deanery; www.nwpgmd.nhs.uk
7   South Yorkshire & South Humber Deanery; www.syshdeanery.com
8   Mersey Deanery; www.merseydeanery.ac.uk
9   Trent Deanery; www.trentdeanery.nottingham.ac.uk
10 West Midlands Deanery; www.wmdeanery.org
11 Leicestershire, Northamptonshire & Rutland Deanery; www.lnrhwd.nhs.uk
12 Eastern Deanery; www.easterndeanery.org
13 Oxford Deanery; www.oxford-pgmde.co.uk
14 London Deanery; www.londondeanery.ac.uk
15 Kent, Surrey & Sussex Deanery; www.kssdeanery.ac.uk
16 Severn & Wessex Deanery; www.sevwesdeanery.nhs.uk
17 South West Peninsula Deanery; www.peninsuladeanery.nhs.uk

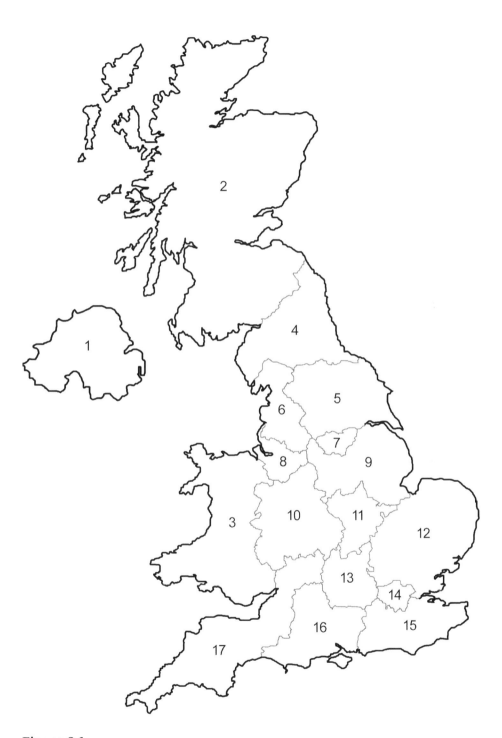

Figure 8.1.

Postscript

The MTAS questions used in 2006/07

The following questions appear on the MTAS application form with a 150 word limit per question, double the 75 word limit of MDAP.

Relevant significant achievement

Give an example of a non-academic achievement explaining both the significance to you and the relevance to foundation training. (6 points)

Academic achievements

List your academic achievements. (4 points)

Dealing effectively with pressure/challenge

Describe an example (not necessarily clinical) of a time when you had to deal with pressure or overcome a setback/challenge. What did you do and what was the outcome? (6 points)

The patient as the central focus of care

Describe an example from your clinical experience where your behaviour enhanced the experience of the patient as the central focus of care. What did you do and what was the outcome? (6 points)

Working effectively with others

Describe an example from your own experience (either clinical or non-clinical) that has increased your understanding of the importance of team working. What was your role and contribution to the team? (6 points)

Professionalism

Describe an example of a situation where you had to demonstrate your professionalism and/or integrity. What did you do and what was the outcome? (6 points)

Organisational skills

Describe an example of how your organisation and planning skills have contributed to a significant personal achievement in the last five years. What did you learn from this which is relevant to foundation training? (6 points)

Index